CANCER ETIOLOGY, DIAGNOSIS AND TREATMENTS

A COMPREHENSIVE TEXTBOOK OF PRIMARY AND METASTATIC SKELETAL SYSTEM TUMORS

Cancer Etiology, Diagnosis and Treatments

Additional books and e-books in this series can be found on Nova's website under the Series tab.

Orthopedic Research and Therapy

Additional books and e-books in this series can be found on Nova's website under the Series tab.

CANCER ETIOLOGY, DIAGNOSIS AND TREATMENTS

A COMPREHENSIVE TEXTBOOK OF PRIMARY AND METASTATIC SKELETAL SYSTEM TUMORS

BABAK OTOUKESH
MEHRDAD BAHRABADI
RAPHAELLE VIALLE
SHAYAN HOSSEINZADEH
FARNOOSH SEDAGHATI
AND
SHAYAN AMIRI

nova
Medicine & Health
New York

Additional color graphics may be available in the e-book version of this book.

Library of Congress Cataloging-in-Publication Data

ISBN: 978-1-53619-104-2

Published by Nova Science Publishers, Inc. † New York

CONTENTS

PREFACE

This book is a comprehensive textbook of primary and metastatic skeletal system tumors which provides the clinical, pathological and imaging data of the skeletal system tumors which is appropriate for all of the clinicians who are practicing in oncology wards, especially Orthopaedic surgeons.

In this book, we discuss the diagnosis and treatment of skeletal system tumors, their clinical signs, and symptoms and we also discuss their pathological aspects of the tumors and we conclude the important images such as plain radiographs, CT scan, MRI, and bone scan.

We tried to bring together the best and the most helpful data of each tumor in order to help the patients and the clinicians of this widespread part of medicine.

ACKNOWLEDGMENT

We would like to express our deep and sincere gratitude to Dr. Hossein Farahini[1], President of Orthopaedics Surgery Ward of Rasoul-E-Akram Hospital, for giving us the opportunity to do research and providing invaluable guidance throughout this research.

We would also like to express our special thanks of gratitude to Dr. Mehdi Moghtadaei[2], Vice Chancellor for International Affairs of Iran University of Medical Sciences. It was a great privilege and honor to work and study under his guidance.

Our sincere thanks also goes to Dr. Ali Yeganeh[3], Associate Professor of Iran University of Medical Sciences. His dynamism, vision, sincerity and motivation have deeply inspired us.

We would also like to extend our gratitude to Dr. Ali Shahsavaripour[4] and Dr. Bahareh Heshmat Ghanderijani[5] and Dr. Amirhosein Meysami[6] for providing us with all the facility was required. Our completion of this project could not have been accomplished without their support.

---

[1] Professor, Department of Orthopaedics Surgery, Rasoul-E-Akram Hospital, Iran University of Medical Sciences , Tehran, Iran.

[2] Professor, Department of Orthopaedics Surgery, Rasoul-E-Akram Hospital, Iran University of Medical Sciences , Tehran, Iran.

[3] Associate Professor, Department of Orthopaedics Surgery, Rasoul-E-Akram Hospital, Iran University of Medical Sciences, Tehran, Iran.

[4] Board certified Orthopaedics surgeon, Iran University of Medical Sciences, Tehran, Iran.

[5] Certified Radiologist, Zahedan University of Medical Sciences, Iran.

[6] Certified Emergency Medicine Specialist, Shahid Beheshty University of Medical Sciences, Tehran, Iran.

ACRONYMS

ABC	Aneurysmal bone cyst
ADC	Apparent diffusion coefficient
AIDS	Acquired immune deficiency Syndrome
AJCC	American Joint Committee on Cancer Staging
ALL	Acute lymphoblastic leukemia
AML	Acute myelogenous leukemia
AP	Anteroposterior
AS	Angiosarcoma
AVN	Avascular necrosis
BS	Bone Scan
BPOP	Bizarre parosteal osteochondromatous proliferation of bone
CBC	Complete blood count
CLL	Chronic lymphocytic leukemia
CML	Chronic myelogenous leukemia
CMF	Chondromyxoid fibroma
CT	Computed tomography
CXR	Chest X-ray
DF	Desmoplastic fibroma
DDx	Differential diagnosis
EIC	Epidermoid inclusion cyst
EG	Eosinophilic granuloma
ESR	Erythrocyte sedimentation rate
ES	Ewing sarcoma
FCD	Fibrous cortical dysplasia
FD	Fibrous dysplasia
FDG	Fluoro-deoxy-glucose
FLAIR	Fluid attenuated inversion recovery
FNA	Fine needle aspiration
FOV	Field of view
FS	Fat-saturated
GCT	Giant cell tumor
G-CSF	Granulocyte colony-stimulating Factor
GI	Gastrointestinal

GY	Gray
HME	Hereditary multiple exostoses
HU	Hounsfield unit
IV	Intravenous
JC	Jaffe–Campanacci syndrome
LCH	Langerhan cell histiocytosis
LSMFT	Liposclerosing myxofibrous tumor
MCL	Medial collateral ligament
MFH	Malignant fibrous histiocytoma
MGUS	Monoclonal gammopathy of undetermined significance
MRA	MR angiography
MRI	Magnetic resonance imaging
NHL	Non-Hodgkin lymphoma
NF1	Neurofibromatosis type 1
NOF	Non-ossifying fibroma
NOS	Not otherwise specified
NSAIDS	Nonsteroidal anti-inflammatory Drug
NSF	Nephrogenic systemic fibrosis
OFD	Osteofibrous dysplasia
PCNB	Percutaneous core needle biopsy
PET	Positron emission tomography
POEMS	Polyneuropathy, organomegaly, endocrinopathy, monoclonal gammopathy
PNET	Primitive neuroectodermal tumor
PSA	Prostate specific antigen
PTH	Parathyroid hormone
PVNS	Pigmented villonodular synovitis
RCC	Renal cell carcinoma
RPMI	Roswell Park Memorial Institute (medium for flow cytometry of lymphoma)
SBC	Simple bone cyst
SBP	Solitary plasmacytoma of bone
SPECT	Single photon emission computed Tomography
SPEP	Serum protein electrophoresis
STIR	Short tau inversion recovery
SUV	Standardized uptake value
T1W	T1-weighted
T2W	T2-weighted
TGFb	Transforming growth factor beta
UPEP	Urine protein electrophoresis
U/S	Ultrasound
VEGF	Vascular endothelial growth factor
WBC	White blood cells
WHO	World Health Organization

Chapter 1

PRINCIPLES OF BONE AND SOFT TISSUE TUMORS

BIOPSY OF MUSCULOSKELETAL TUMORS

- According to Jaffe in 1958, a biopsy is the final step in achieving a diagnosis, not a shortcut.
- In the past, the importance of the inaccurate biopsy, which was often associated with significant contamination of the surrounding soft tissue, was insignificant, since most malignant tumors were treated with amputation.
- Today, organ preservation procedures can be performed on 90 to 95% of musculoskeletal tumors. Therefore, the method of biopsy should allow the maintenance of the limb.
- Biopsies should be performed on malignant, benign aggressive lesions and radiographically-suspicious lesions.

BIOLOGY OF MUSCULOSKELETAL TUMORS

- Sarcomas (bone, soft tissue) tend to grow from center towards periphery, meaning that the newest part of the tumor is the periphery.
- The peripheral reactive zone includes mesenchymal cells, angiogenesis, and inflammatory process.
- Type of proliferation differs, depending on the location of the lesion:
  - Soft tissue tumors have a fibrotic tissue reaction.
  - Bone tumors have a sclerotic bone reaction.
  - According to this principle, even a single lesion in different zones induces different reactive mesenchymal responses:
  - In the intraosseous zone: reactive sclerotic
  - In soft tissue components: fibrotic tissue reaction
- Unlike sarcomas, carcinomas usually infiltrate healthy tissue instead of pushing it around, and usually do not produce a reactive zone.
- Satellites: are nodular tumors invaded to the peripheral reactive zone, not metastases.

- Skip lesions: are nodular tumors outside the reactive zone but inside that very anatomic compartment and are only seen in high-grade sarcomas.
- Bone and soft tissue tumors initially metastasize to lungs and then to other bones.

Anatomic Location of Biopsy Tract

- In musculoskeletal tumors, and because of regional morphologic variations, multiple specimens are needs for the diagnosis to be confirmed.
- In carcinomas, and because of its homogeneity, one core biopsy specimen or tissue aspiration is sufficient for confirmation of the diagnosis.
- Biopsy errors are defined as incorrect or inconclusive diagnosis secondary to biopsy not from the primary lesion.
- Two questions need to be answered:
  1) What region of the lesion should be biopsied?
  2) What is the most harmless anatomic path to reach the lesion?
- There is no definitive objective evidence supporting growth acceleration or metastatic spread of the lesion after the biopsy.
- The actual risk of open or fine needle biopsy is the local spread of the tumor and the facilitation of its local relapse. The risk seems to be higher in open biopsy than a fine needle biopsy, in non-hemostatic than hemostatic procedures, and in wider biopsy tracts than narrower ones. Therefore, in the restoration of the biopsy wound, it is recommended to keep the sutures as close to the cutting edge of the skin as possible.
- The practitioner performing the biopsy must be informed about the final surgical technique.
- It will be best if the patients' therapist is the practitioner who performs the biopsy.

Principles

- Extra-osseous components of bone tumors are representative of the tumor as much as intra-osseous components and if exists, should be biopsied while the cortex remains intact.
- Drain insertion site should be along the main incisional site.
- The biopsy tract should reach the tumor via the shortest path, not contaminate more than one compartment and stay far away from neurovascular structures as much as possible.

Biopsy Techniques

- An open incisional biopsy allows evaluation of cell morphology, tissue structure, IHC, cytogenic, flow-cytometry, and electron microscopy.

- In a fine needle biopsy, not enough tissue is sampled from the tissue cortex and therefore the tumor structure is not visualized, so FNA has no role in primary bone tumors.
- CNB: using a 14G needle provides a cylinder of tissue with a maximum length of 20mm.
- More than 90% accuracy in differentiation of malignant VS benign lesions.
- In most soft tissue and bone tumors, a biopsy is a choice before therapy commencement.
- An open biopsy is performed only in cases with vague pathology results.
- A biopsy should be performed under the guidance of CT or C-arm.
- Multiple core specimens must be sampled.
- In deeply located tumors, a biopsy must be performed under the guidance of CT.

Principles of Incisional Biopsy

- The shortest possible longitudinal incision is used to obtain a sufficient specimen. Transverse incisions should be avoided.
- Use a knife or curette to prevent the specimen tissue from being crushed.
- In bone, an oval cavity with a round margin should be used.
- A tiny hole is preferred for biopsy, unless a larger specimen is needed, in which a rectangular hole is used.
- Always send a sample for frozen-section to ensure that there is enough tissue specimen representing the tumor.
- In case a live tumor cell is not detected, biopsy should be repeated.
- Culture on the biopsy sample and biopsy on cultured specimens should always be performed.
- Precise hemostasis is essential. Large hematomas may contaminant the whole organ, making organ salvage impossible.
- A tourniquet is rarely used in the biopsy. In the case of utilization, an Esmarch bandage should not be used for evacuation of blood from muscle.
- Tourniquet should be deflated before wound closure.
- Drains is inserted if needed.
- The drain should come out from one of the ends along the incision, not next to it.

Principles of Radiotherapy

Radiotherapy has two mechanisms of action:

1) Production of free intracellular free radicals
2) Direct genetic damage by them

Cells' sensitivity to radiotherapy depends on:

1) The phase of cell in the meiosis cycle. Cells in active division phase are more sensitive to radiotherapy.
2) Tissue oxygenation. Local hypoxia has a protective effect against radiotherapy because free radicals are not produced in this environment.
3) The cell's ability to repair DNA damage or its inability to enter apoptosis in response to radiotherapy-induced damage.

INDICATIONS

In Absolute Control of Tumor (Primary Malignant Bone Tumors)

1) Ewing sarcoma/ PNET
2) Lymphoma
3) Hemangioendothelioma
4) Solitary *plasmacytoma of bone*

As Adjuvant Therapy

In Soft tissue sarcomas, may be given before or after surgery, however does not make a difference in overall survival.

As Palliative Care

1) In metastatic bone disease.
2) After fixation of pathologic/impending fractures, in order to reduce the overall volume of the tumor

Prostate tumors are highly sensitive to radiation.
Breast tumors are 70% sensitive to radiation.
Renal and gastric tumors are radiation-resistant.

TECHNIQUE

1 rad: 1 centigray
1 gray: 1 joule of absorbed energy per tissue kilogram
The typical dose is 150-200 rod/day
Radiation is given
The radiation is given in splits because of its cumulative effects.

The total dose of radiation is the sum of all daily doses. For myeloma, it is 30-40 gray and for soft tissue sarcoma, up to 60 grays.

Total Dose

>4500 rad: no effect on wound repair
4500 -5500 rad: tissue repairs but with side effects
<6000 rad: tissue is not healed

Tumors' Sensitivity to Radiotherapy

Most of the primary bone malignancies are radiotherapy-resistant. Sensitive tumors are:

- Multiple myeloma
- Lymphoma
- Ewing sarcoma

Metastatic bone carcinoma, except for renal cell carcinoma, are sensitive to radiotherapy. It is used for reducing the chance of relapse, after marginal resection of malignant soft tissue tumors, and as an alternative for extensive surgeries or amputation.

Pre-operative radiotherapy of soft tissue sarcomas is used for reducing the tumor volume, making its resection easier.

It is rarely used for benign lesions:

- Extensive PVNS
- Massive GCT in spine

SIDE EFFECTS

Acute

Skin irritation is the most common adverse effect. Initial erythema may lead to .... Especially in those under cytotoxic therapy.

Gastric side effects
Frequency
Fatigue
Lack of appetite
Limb edema

Late

Chronic edema
Fibrosis
Joint stiffness

Osteonecrosis
Pathologic fractures
It has become increasingly prevalent and treatment could be hard.

- 47% in female with the above-mentioned treatment
- 66% in female with the above-mentioned treatment plus chemotherapy

Pediatric-Specific Complications

Scoliosis
Kyphosis
Deformity of thorax
Ilium hypoplasia
Limb length difference due to physeal arrest

Malignancy Development to Secondary Sarcoma

It has become increasingly prevalent,
Almost 10 years after radiotherapy.
Prognosis is poor.
Even more prevalent in patients undergoing chemotherapy.

Techniques of Radiotherapy

- The conventional method with external radiation.
- Brachytherapy (close-up radiation)
- Catheters are placed in the tumor bed at the time of resection. The other end of the catheter is out of the skin.
- Allows delivering a higher dose of radiation to the target tissue.
- At the edge of the radiotherapy field, the radiation dose is drastically reduced, reducing damage to healthy tissue.
- Infection and delayed wound healing are among the side effects.

Chemotherapy

Principles

Using new chemotherapy regimens, the 5-year survival of patients with osteosarcoma and Ewing sarcoma is about 70%. Chemotherapy has an effective role in the treatment of MFH and childhood high-grade sarcomas (i.e., RMS). In most adult soft tissue malignancies, chemotherapy does not have a role, making only a slight improvement in the outcome. Chemotherapy is useless in most of the low-grade and cartilage tumors.

TYPES

Adjuvant: Chemotherapy that is delivered after surgery, aiming to destroy micro-metastases.

Neo-adjuvant: chemotherapy that is delivered before surgery.

Pros and Cons

- Neo-adjuvant chemotherapy reduces the bulk of the tumor, making limb salvage surgery easier.
- Allow histological evaluation of chemotherapy effect on tumor cells. This is called necrosis percentage and is one of the most valuable prognostic factors.
- Histologic evaluation of chemotherapy effect allow changing the regiments, in case the current one is not effective.
- Theoretically, reduces the spread of tumor cells during surgery.
- Starting chemotherapy before surgery, and as soon as the diagnosis is confirmed, (lung) micro-metastases are treated. Otherwise, during the recovery period after surgery and until the patient is ready for chemotherapy (almost 3 weeks), the treatment of micrometastases is delayed.
- Provides the possibility of designing a custom implant for the patient without delay in treatment.
- Gives the patient and his/her family the opportunity to choose amputation or limb salvage.
- Some believe that increases the risk of infection and delayed wound healing.

TECHNIQUE

- 3-4 weeks after the last dose of chemotherapy, surgery is performed.
- Adjuvant chemotherapy, starting at least two weeks post-operatively due to wound healing process.

METHOD OF CHEMOTHERAPY

Using multiple agents: Different cells of the tumor use different defense mechanism. To overcome this issue, multiple agents are used.

Chemotherapy Side Effects

- Alkylating agents: Mustards

Cyclophosphamide: hemorrhagic cystitis, leukopenia, alopecia
Ifosfamide: hemorrhagic cystitis

- Platinum compounds

Cisplatin: nephrotoxicity (Cumulative and irreversible), ototoxicity (Cumulative and irreversible), peripheral neuropathy (reversible)
Carboplatin: nephrotoxicity, myelosuppression

- Anti-metabolites

Methotrexate: myelosuppression, hepatotoxicity, pneumonitis

- Anti-tumors antibiotics

Doxorubicin: myelosuppression, acute and chronic cardio toxicity, severe tissue necrosis in case of extravasation
Dactinomycin: myelosuppression, severe tissue necrosis in case of extravasation, N&V, diarrhea

- Epipodophyllotoxins

Etoposide: mucositis, N&V

- Anti-microtubules

Vinca alkaloids
Vincristine: peripheral neuropathy (irreversible), tissue necrosis in case of extravasation, alopecia

Cryosurgery

Definition

Using extreme cold to kill tumor cells

MECHANISM

Immediate Cell Necrosis

- Crystallization and rupturing the cell membrane (main mechanism)
- Making thermal shock
- Intra-cellular dehydration due to the shift of water towards extra-cellular crystallization, and consequent electrolyte imbalance
- Denaturation of cell proteins

Late Cell Necrosis

- Micro-vascular circulation disorder
- Vascular stasis

PATHOPHYSIOLOGY

- Following immediate crystallization (for example after using liquid nitrogen), extra and intracellular fluids are crystalized.
- Following gradual crystallization, the first extra cellular and then intracellular fluids are crystalized.
- Following gradual warming, intracellular fluid is re-crystallized and therefore the cell membrane is ruptured.
- Following immediate warming, unlike gradual warming, cell membrane rupture does not happen.
- Therefore, the most damage to a living cell is when it is crystallized immediately and warmed gradually, which is exacerbated by repeating the cycles.

HISTORY

The effects of liquid nitrogen on normal animal bone were first investigated by Gage in 1966. It was in those years that researchers found that -21 to -60 degrees Celsius was sufficient for tissue necrosis and that greater coldness did not produce more lethality.

CLINICAL APPLICATION

Invasive Benign Tumors

- GCT
- ABC

- UBC
- FD
- Enchondroma
- Chondroblastoma
- Eosinophilic granuloma
- Osteoblastoma
- Chondromyxoid fibroma

Malignant Tumors

- Low grade chondrosarcoma
- Metastatic tumors

Types of Cryosurgery

Direct Application of Liquid Nitrogen

A tourniquet is used to keep the field free of blood and to prevent the warming effects of blood, which prevents cryotherapy. After extensive tumor curettage, possible holes in the remaining cavity of the tumor are closed with gel foam to prevent fluid nitrogen from spreading to surrounding healthy tissue. A thermocouple is used to record the temperature of the tumor cavity, its wall, and surrounding tissue. The surrounding soft tissue is washed with warm saline while pouring liquid nitrogen into the tumor cavity to prevent them from becoming cold. Cryosurgery begins with the addition of liquid nitrogen and lasts for 1 to 2 minutes. Spontaneous warm-up takes 3 to 5 minutes. When the cavity temperature reaches above zero degrees, the cycle ends. This cycle is repeated twice. The tumor cavity is then flushed with normal saline and ready to either be filled with cement or receive a bone graft.

Argon Gas Technique

After extensive tumor curettage, the cavity is filled with a gel. This gel acts as a thermal conductor and sticks to all parts of the cavity, due to its adhesion potentiality. Argon gas is introduced into the cavity by metal probes embedded in the gel. Due to the adhesion potentiality of the gel, all parts of the cavity are evenly cooled. The computer controls the delivery of argon gas until it reaches the desired temperature.

Post-Cryosurgery Care

- Prophylactic antibiotics are prescribed for 3 to 5 days after surgery.
- In lower limb lesions, the patient should avoid weight-bearing activities for 6 weeks.

- After this period, a control radiograph is taken and if the healing process is satisfactory, Partial weighing bearing starts.

Complications

- Fracture: It is considered pathological after cryosurgery because it has happened in a cold-weekend bone.
- These fractures tend to heal slowly (mean 3 to 9 months).
- Late weighting and use of internal fixation with cement prevent pathological fractures to a large extent
- Nerve paresis: is usually transient and resolves on its own.
- Adjacent cartilage damage: is rare and is seen in less than 3% of cases.
- Gas embolism: is very rare and only four cases have been reported. Most of the nitrogen used in the cold process turn into bubbles and comes out of the wound. It rarely enters the blood-circulation and lungs.
- It is seen as a drop in oxygen saturation, a decrease in blood pressure, an increase in heart rate. It is managed by discontinuing NO and delivering oxygen.

Results

Using this method to treat benign invasive tumors makes the rate of recurrence less than 5%.

Photodynamic Treatment of Tumors

Definition

- Administration of a non-toxic drug called photosensitizer systemically, locally or topically to the tumor site.

Mechanism of Action

- Following administration, the drug accumulates in the tumor tissue.
- Applying light to the tumor site makes cytotoxic substances and induces necrosis of tumor cells.
- Oxygen must be available in the environment for this method to work.

History

- First discovered by a medical student in Munich named Oscar Rabb in 1900.

Clinical Application

- 5-amino-levulinic acid (5-ALA) is under study in the treatment of desmoid tumor.
- In a desmoid tumor, a positive margin is strongly associated with the likelihood of tumor recurrence.
- Administration causes Protoporphyrin IX (PPIX).
- It is administrated three hours before the operation.
- Protoporphyrin IX (PPIX) receives pink fluorescence under blue light. This fluorescence is seen in the macroscopic sample of the tumor, although microscopic remnants of the tumor at the surgical site might not be detected this way due to a small size.

Protoporphyrin IX (PPIX) is cytotoxic if under red light for 30 minutes. It is irradiated to the tumor bed to remove the microscopic remnants of the tumor, if any.

Chapter 2

BENIGN TUMORS

OSTEOID OSTEOMA

Definition

- A benign tumor consists of an osteoblast mass called nidus that is surrounded by reactive sclerosis of the surrounding bone.

Epidemiology

- Maximum prevalence is in the age of 5 to 25 years. 80% of cases are at this age. It has a peak age in the second decade.
- It is twice as common in men as in women.
- It accounts for 3% of all bone tumors, and 12% of benign bone tumors.

Source

- Osteoblastic neoplasms with connective tissue are very bloody.

Location

- In order of prevalence: femur + tibia 60%, spine (posterior element 90%), hand (p1 & metacarpus), foot (talus).
- In the upper limb, the most common site is in the distal humerus near the elbow.
- Not reported in the skull, sternum, and clavicle.
- It can be spatial, cortical, medullary, or subperiosteal.
- The most common site is intracortical.

Signs

- It is rare in the pineal gland and can lead to joint swelling, joint dryness, and bone growth disorders.
- In spine, it can cause scoliosis, which is painful as; lumbar spine is more common than other affected areas. On the concave side, there is a deviation of the spine.
- It is always painful. The pain is more severe at night.
- If there is no pain, another diagnosis should be considered. Except for the osteoid osteoma of the hand, which can be painless.
- Tenderness is a pointed sign of osteoid osteoma, nerve tumors, and tumor glomus. In the lower extremities, it is often accompanied by lameness. In cases of long term disease, muscle atrophy has been seen. Decreased deep tendon reflexes have also been observed.
- Causes symptoms of arthritis when it is close to the joint. Symptoms include muscle atrophy, joint dryness, deformity, and synovial hypertrophy.
- In small bones, limbs are associated with increased local growth
- When it starts at the age of less than 5 years, it can cause a difference in limb length by stimulating the growth of the affected limb.
- The cause of pain is PG release (PGE2, Prostacyclin). Painless lesions are often in hand.

Imaging

- It is 80% cortical.
- Typically, the diaphysis involves long bones
- Nidus is Lucent. Inside it, calcification may be seen.
- The reaction of the surrounding healthy tissue is sclerotic.
- If it is inside the medullary canal, pericardial, or subperiosteal, there is no surrounding sclerosis.

CT

- The best modality to detect Nidus.
- Nidus may be mineralized in the center in various forms (50% Mineralized items)
- Be sure to ask for one-millimeter cuts and Bone window to find Nidus.

MRI

- Nidus (high T2، low T1) Often is not seen.
- In cases where the nidus is inside the medullary canal, periarticular, or subperiosteal, there is no surrounding sclerosis. In these cases, the accuracy of CT scan is low because the contrast between the Nidus radio center and the surrounding bone is low, and therefore MRI is helpful.
- Due to edema adjacent to the surrounding bone marrow, it may be confused with aggressive lesions.

BS

- Increases absorption in all three phases.
- If osteoids are suspected but are not seen on the radiograph, the next step is to perform a bone scan to determine the extent of the lesion. Then we perform a CT scan of that area to see Nidus.
- Double density sign: The absorption of radioactive material in the center is more than the environment.

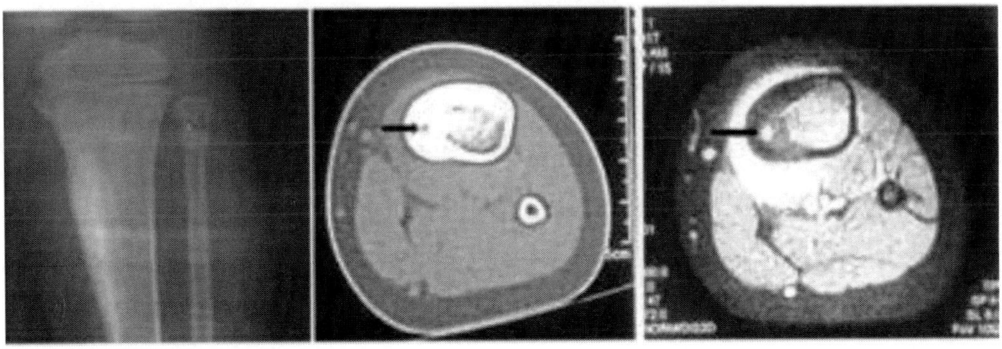

Figure 2-1. Osteoid osteoma of proximal tibia in a 5 year old boy X-ray, CT scan and MRI.

Macroscopic Pathology

- It is a red circular or oval area that is easily distinguished from adjacent areas.
- Around Nidus, there is a large area of sclerotic bone.
- Tetracycline labeling, Helps to find Nidus before the operation. During operation, Nidus is distinguished from the surrounding sclerotic bone under fluorescent light.
- In this method, tetracycline is administered for the patient one to two days before the operation, then during the operation, the tumor is examined with an ultraviolet lamp after the operating room light is dimmed to find the tumor. In children under eight years, it can cause permanent discoloration of the teeth and therefore it is not used.

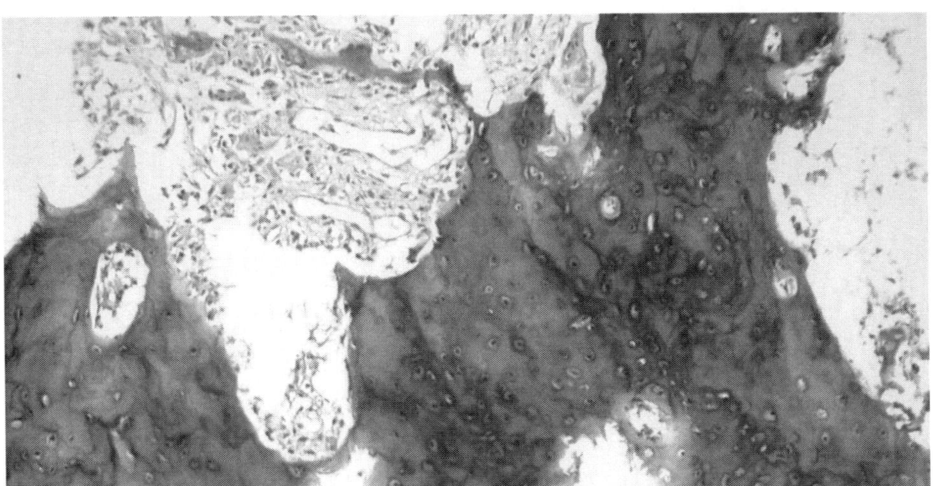

Figure 2-2. Osteoid osteoma: Bone trabeculae are located inside loose vascular connective tissue.

Microscopic Pathology

- Bone trabeculae are located inside loose vascular connective tissue.

Treatment

- Spontaneous healing is reported, probably due to infarction of Nidus.
- NSAIDS
- Excision
- Surgery is used in cases where Nidus is 1.5 cm away from important neurovascular structures, or if other treatments fail. During surgery to reach the nidus, it is best to remove the bone cortex using a high-speed milling machine. The risk of pathological fracture in this method is less than using an osteotomy.
- (Radio Frequency Ablation): Although in the spine use RFA Theoretically, it can be associated with the risk of nerve damage, but to date, many cases of osteoarthritis of the spine have been treated in this way without neurological problems. There is no place in the hand due to the possibility of thermal necrosis. It is widely used and successfully in other areas. Recurrence is 10%. A CT scan under the guidance probe is inserted into Nidus and 90 ° C is applied for 6 minutes.
- (MRgFUs) Magnetic resonance-guided focused ultrasound: In this method, with the help of MRI to guide the ultrasound waves and monitor the heat caused by them, these waves are concentrated inside Nidus so that Nidus disappears with the resulting heat. The advantage of this method is that it does not use radiation.
- Has no potential for malignancy

Differential Diagnosis

- Stress Fracture: In radiographs, lucency is linear and perpendicular to the surface of the cortex.
- Brodie abscess: It is intramedullary. There may be an infection of the sinus tract. There is severe edema around the lesion.
- Laboratory tests help to differentiate Indus.
- Osteoblastoma: It is more common in Spine. Nidus is larger than 1.5 to 2 cm.
- Osteosarcoma: The soft tissue component is more invasive and larger.
- Osteoma: It has no nidus, no increase in absorption on bone scan, and no edema on MRI.
- Bone Island: No nidus, no increase in bone resorption, and no MRI edema.
- Chondroblasts: Epiphyseal and intra-medullary.

OSTEOMA

Definition

- It is not a neoplasm but a thickened Hamartoma of the cortical bone.

Epidemiology

- It is common in the fourth and fifth decades
- F > M

Location

- It is 70%present in the frontal sinuses. It is generally seen in the skull and sinuses.
- The sphenoid lesion is associated with Gardner syndrome.

Clinical Signs

- It is asymptomatic.
- Rarely, when it is in the inner table of the skull, it has neurological symptoms.
- Infection can be caused by sinus obstruction.
- There is a vision problem in the orbital type.

Imaging

- It is on the surface of the bone and is very dense.
- The margin of the lesion is perfectly smooth and clear from the surroundings.
- No modular canal.
- Low signal in all MRI sequences

BS

- Usually not absorbed. If active, the absorption is slight.

Treatment

- Should be excised if symptomatic.

BONE ISLAND (B.I)

Definition

- Is a hamartoma (normal tissue located in an abnormal location).

Epidemiology

- Very common. It is discovered by chance.
- M = F.

Common Place

- It is a peri-articular and can be anywhere on the skeleton.
- In the pelvis, the proximal femur and ribs are most common. It is rare in the spine.

Imaging

- Oval-shaped with a distinguished border.
- The size is typically less than 1 cm.
- The giant type is larger than 2 cm.
- The longitudinal axis is parallel to the long bones.
- Brush border with radial spicules in the margin.
- It is uniformly dense.

MRI

- Has a low signal in all sequences.
- No surrounding edema (differentiation from sclerotic metastasis).

BS

- It usually does not increase absorption. Large and metabolically active lesions can increase absorption.

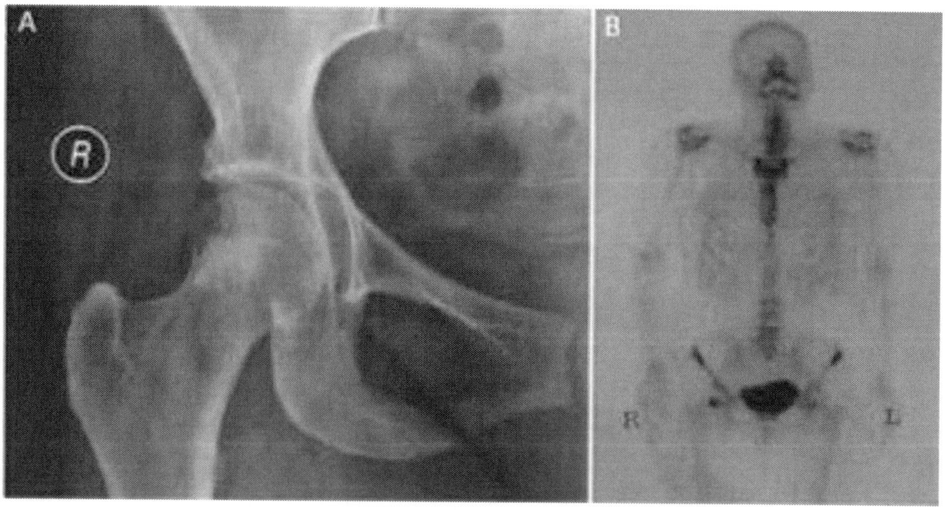

Figure 2-3. Bone Island in bone scan (right) and Xray (left).

Treatment

- If the lesion grows (more than 25 percent in six months or 50 percent in twelve months) a biopsy should be done.
- Has no potential for malignancy. It can spontaneously grow, shrink, or disappear.

Differential Diagnosis

- Sclerotic metastasis: No radial spicules. There is edema around.
- Low-grade osteosarcoma: Usually larger than Bone island.
- Melorheostosis: has a candle wax dripping appearance.
- Bone Island: There are several osteopoikilosis in the pelvis or shoulder girdle.
- Osteopathia striata.
- AD.
- It has a fan-like appearance of sclerosis in the long bones and pelvis.
- Osteoid Osteoma: Typically cortical.

Osteochondroma

Definition

- In the past, it was considered an evolutionary anomaly that led to exophytic growth at the bone surface.
- EXT1 and EXT2 are currently considered real tumors due to their association with the genes.

Epidemiology

- The most common tumor is a bone lesion. It exists in 3% of the population.
- 30-50% of benign bone lesions.
- M =1.8 F.
- All patients are less than 30 years old at the time of initial diagnosis. The peak age of diagnosis is the second decade.

Common Places

- Metaphysial or metadiaphysial in long bones. It is more common in femoral TB and humerus.
- 35% are seen around the knee. Then in the proximal femur and proximal humerus.
- It is more common in the ilium and scapula than the broad bone group.
- Rare in the spine. Not seen in craniofacial.

Clinical Symptoms

- Hard swelling has been the most common symptom for many years. The symptoms are mostly mechanical.
- Paresthesia or pseudoaneurysm can be seen due to pressure on the neurovascular. Pseudoendrism is typically in the popliteal.
- Osteochondroma fracture.
- Bursitis Bursa on the tumor.
- Decreased range of motion.
- Cord compression if it is close to the spinal cord. Progressive lower limb weakness in an exoskeleton patient is indicated by MRI examination of the spine to diagnose extradural exostosis.

Imaging

- The bone marrow and cortex are lesions along the bone marrow and the main bone cortex.
- The base of the exostosis is often located away from the nearest joint due to the pressure of the surrounding muscles.
- The cartilaginous cap is thicker in children.
- Cap> 2 cm in adults and Cap> 3 cm in children suspected of malignancy.
- By comparison, the average Cap thickness in chondrosarcoma is 5 to 6 cm.
- CT to measure Cap thickness may be unreliable.
- Ultrasound is suitable for measuring Cap thickness but is incapable of deep lesions.
- MRI is the best means of measuring cartilage cap. In T2, it is clear due to a large amount of water in the hyaline cartilage.
- There may be a bursa on the tumor. Inside the bursa, the buccal synovial signal may increase and, if synovial, chondromatosis may occur. In calcified T2 chondromatosis, there are signs of signal reduction.

The Potential for Malignancy

- Less than 1% has been reported in the single type.
- 3 to 5% in hereditary multipurpose exudative malignancies. In other reports, 5-25% has been reported.
- The above was about becoming chondrosarcoma. It can also lead to Osteosarcoma, which is less common.
- An increase in cap thickness or a change in the orientation of calcifications, especially after puberty, should be associated with suspected malignancy. Malignancy should be suspected when a previous benign tumor suddenly develops in an adult. If malignancy is suspected, the lesion is completely removed and its prognosis is good. A biopsy is not indicated in these cases because it may not be removed from the malignant area and is misleading.

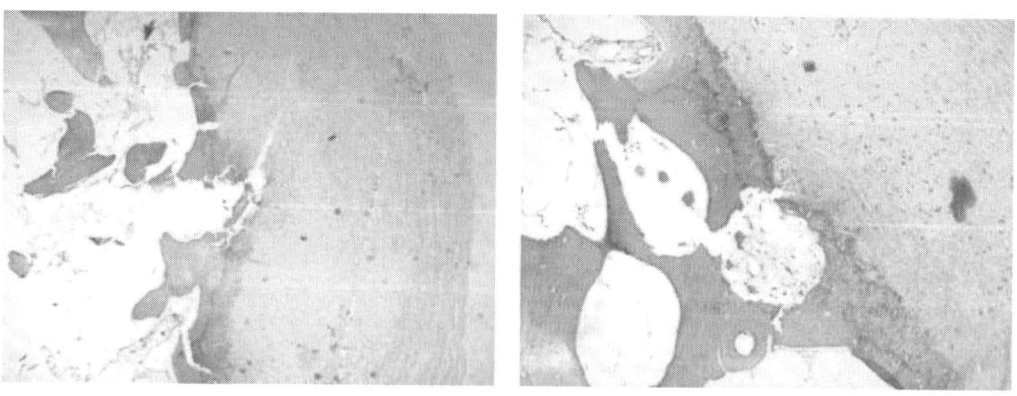

Figure 2-4. Osteochondroma: Lubricated cartilaginous cap lined with perichondrium. The perichondrium is along the periosteum of the main bone. The cap is made of hyaline cartilage and is usually 2 to 10 mm thick.

Macroscopic Pathology

- Lubricated cartilaginous cap lined with perichondrium. The perichondrium is along the periosteum of the main bone.
- The cap is made of hyaline cartilage and is usually 2 to 10 mm thick.
- Microscopic pathology.
- The cartilaginous cap is covered with medium cellular hyaline cartilage.

Treatment

- Follow-up for large lesions is recommended by radiography. They are often not surgically removed until they become symptomatic or malignant. These include symptomatic pressure on the neurovascular, joint dysfunction, and cosmetic problems for the patient. Recurrence is about 2%. If surgery is needed, it is better to wait until skeletal maturity, because then the risk of recurrence and damage to the pharynx is lower.

Other

- The most common benign tumor is associated with radiotherapy.
- Differential Diagnosis.
- Osi-fican myositis: Separated from the bone.
- Parosteal osteosarcoma: The medullary and cortical parts of the tumor are not along the medulla and cortex of the main bone.
- Trever Discasc (Hemiplicular Epiphyseal Splasia): Osteochondromas originate in the epiphyseal articular cartilage, are intra-articular, are often found in the lower extremities, especially the distal femur, proximal tia, talus, and navicular, and are associated with variation in limb length. In case of multi-joint conflict, it tends to be one-sided.
- Bizarre parosteal osteochondromatous proliferation, BPOP (Noras's lesion): superficial lesion including bone and cartilage originate from periostum.

HME (Hereditary Multiple Exostosis)

- Autosomal dominant.
- In the male sex, it is seen twice as much as the female sex.
- With or without a base.
- Short stature is seen due to stunted growth.
- They have skeletal deformity due to growth disorders. This deformity in the upper limb is shortening of the ulna and the radius is arch-shaped, which may lead to radial head dislocation. Synostosis of the radius and ulna may also be seen. Forearm deformity is a cosmetic problem in these patients that can be treated with osteotomies. Radial head dislocation can be resected if it is symptomatic after puberty. Radius and ulna synostosis is usually not a major problem for the patient. Removing the radius exostosis has been shown to prevent the progression of forearm deformity. In severe forearm deformity, the formation of a forearm bone is helpful. In the lower extremities,

the genus Valgus is common and it originates from proximal tibial. Severe deformity can be treated with epiphysiodesis before puberty. After skeletal maturation, genuvalgus can be treated by proximal tibia osteotomies but if there is exostosis of the fibula head, osteotomy can lead to peroneal nerve palsy. Ankle valgus is also seen, which is recommended to correct the tibial angle.

- Most are baseless. The lesions are larger than the single type.
- Becoming malignant occurs at a younger age than the single type.
- Nuclear scans and baseline radiographs are recommended in areas where we have difficulty diagnosing physical examination.
- Lesions are followed up every 2-3 years by radiography. Symptomatic lesions fall off sooner.
- They occur at a younger age than the singular type and the average age of diagnosis is three years old (due to the presence of bony prominences, or deformity or different lengths of limbs).
- The prevalence of HME-affected areas is similar to their frequency in the individual type.
- The most common site of involvement is around the knee. Ninety-four percent are likely to have distal femur, proximal tibia, or proximal fibula, so a knee radiograph is a good screening test.

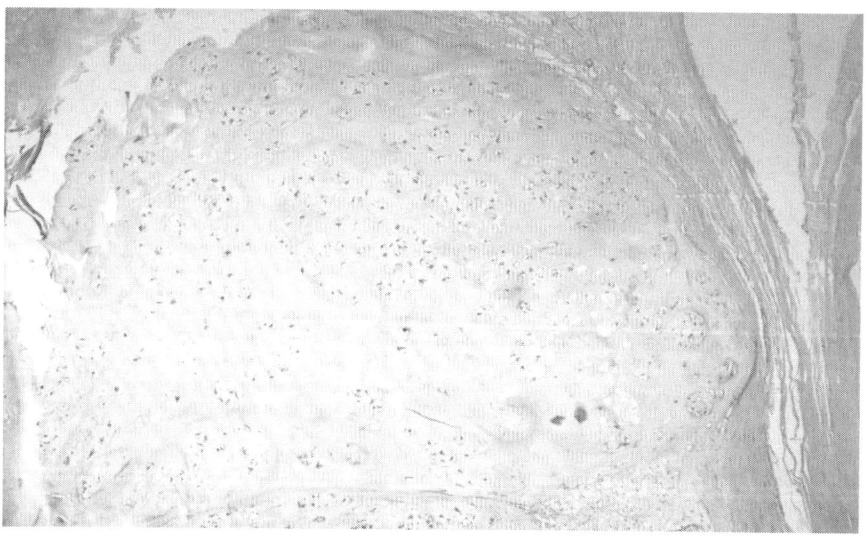

Figure 2-5. Exostosis.

Suspected Malignancy in Osteochondroma

- Increase in cartilaginous capsize after skeletal maturation.
- Cap greater than 2 cm (adults) or 3 cm (children).
- Areas of lucency within the lesion.
- Cortical destruction of the main bone.
- Large soft tissue mass with scattered and irregular calcification.
- Change in the orientation of calcification.

ENCHONDROMA

Definition

- Benign neoplasm is a common intramodular neoplasm composed of mature cartilage.
- Epidemiology.
- The second to fourth decades of age are common. The peak age of diagnosis is thirty-five years old.
- F = M.
- It accounts for 10 to 25% of all benign bone tumors.

Common Place

- The tubular bones of the hands and feet make up a total of 60% of cases. The hand is seven times more common than the foot. The most common bone tumor is the hand.
- Long bones are the second most common. The femur is the most common of these. The distal femur accounts for 20% and the proximal arm for 10%.

Clinical Signs

- Mostly discovered by accident.
- Pathological fracture.
- Painful lesions should arouse suspicion of malignant degeneration.

Imaging

- A geographic lesion with calcification in the form of arcs & rings.
- Can be stretched in the hands and feet. The entire bone shaft can be involved in the fingers.
- Typically central is metaphysical.
- Endosteal scalloping may be present due to lobular growth but should be less than 2/3 of the thickness of the cortex.
- It is mistaken for bone infarct but there is no expansion in the latter case, and the margin of the lesion is quite sharp and jagged.

CT

- The degree of endosteal scalloping and occult fracture is accurately indicated.

MRI

- T1 has a dark signal (due to abundant water in the hyaline cartilage).
- T2 has a clear signal (due to abundant water in the hyaline cartilage).

- Signalvoid calcification can distort the clear signal in the tumor.
- Artifacts around the lesion can be seen due to the interference of the abundant water signal inside the lesion with the fat bone signal of the surrounding bone marrow.
- More than 90% of bone marrow filling on MRI by a cartilaginous tumor suggests chondrosarcoma.

BS

- It is Hot or Warm.
- It is useful in finding multiple lesions.

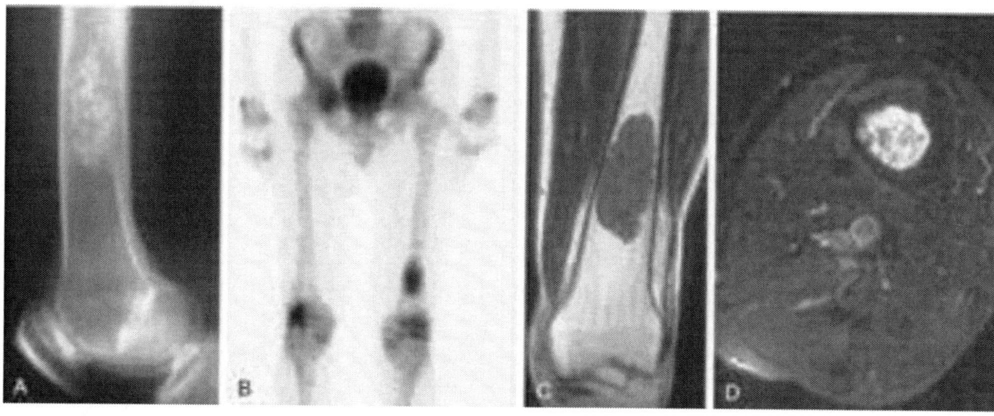

Figure 2-6. Popcorn view in x-ray (A). Increase in uptake in bone scan (B). T1 fat suppress MRI shows low signal (c) and T2 fat suppress MRI shows high signal (D).

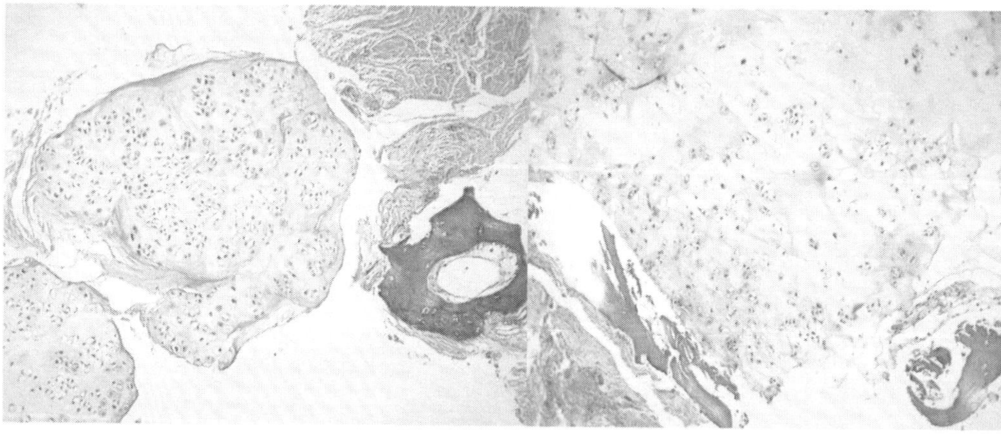

Figure 2–7. Enchondroma: Lobules of hyaline cartilage encased by bone and covered by perichondrium.

The Potential for Malignancy

- Less than 1% in single lesions

Treatment

- Follow-up especially for large lesions. Every 3 to 6 months for 1 to 2 years, then annually.
- Cone graft curettage for suspected or large lesions prone to fracture, or observation of changes in serial radiographs.
- Immobilization and subsequent curettage with bone grafts: for pathological fractures.
- Recurrence is rare.

Other

- It is more likely to be lytic in the limbs and occurs with a pathological fracture.
- The most common benign bone tumor is in the hand.

DD

- Low-grade chondrosarcoma: Endosteal scalloping, bone destruction, and more soft tissue component.
- Bone infract calcification: There is a perpendicular serpentine without bone dilatation, and without a central cartilage case.

Low Grade Chondrosarcoma

- Endosteal scalloping should be more than 2.3 times the thickness of the cortex (what is the best radiological distinction).
- Pain, especially in the lesion without previous pain.
- Growing lesion (especially after skeletal puberty).
- Periosteal reaction.
- Axial lesions (pelvis, scapula, and sternum) are more likely to be malignant.
- Larger than 5 cm The size of most enchondromas is three to four cm in size
- Soft tissue component.
- More than 90% of bone marrow filling on MRI by a cartilaginous tumor suggests chondrosarcoma.
- Epiphyseal position.
- Lucent areas within the lesion are highly calcified (biopsy of these areas should be performed).
- Absorption intensity in BS is higher than the anterior cortex of the ilium.

Multiple Enchondromatosis (ME) Including Ollier and Maffucci

- It is congenital but not inherited unlike HME.
- Lesions stop growing at skeletal maturity, but stunted growth and deformity usually occur in the diseased limb at that time. Knee deformity in these patients is genovarum and is the main source of distal femoral deformity.
- Often on one side of the body. One-sidedness can cause a difference in length about ten to twenty-five centimeters of the lower limbs until puberty. The hands are mostly

affected. Cartilaginous columns with fan-like septations are seen instead of round or oval shapes that occur in a single type (Fluted column sign).

- 10 to 25% become chondrosarcomas even in the hand. 25 to 30% in some reports.
- In Maffucci syndrome, there is lateral cavernous hemangioma (phlebitis on radiography).
- Maffucci syndrome has a higher risk of malignancy than Ollier. 25 to 100% risk of malignancy is seen. An increased risk of astrocytoma and gastrointestinal malignancies has also been observed.

METACHONDROMATOSIS

- It is enchondromatosis and osteochondromatosis together.
- Unlike non-hereditary Ollier, this disease is predominantly autosomal recessive, with incomplete penetration.
- Enchondromas affect the iliac crest and metaphyses of long bones
- Osteochondromatic lesions affect most of the hands.
- So far, two cases of metachondromatosis turning into chondrosarcoma have been reported in the world, the second case has been reported by the author.

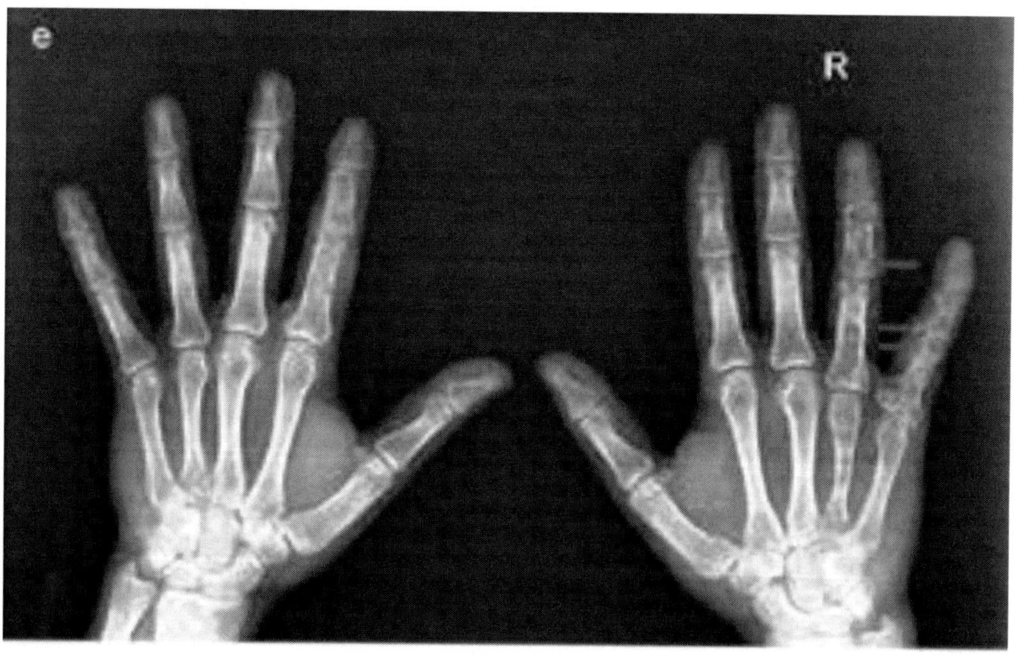

Figure 2-8. Metachondromatosis.

Periosteal Chondroma

Source

- Benign lesion of the cartilage at the surface of the periosteum that resembles an endchroma histologically epidemiologically.
- Age is common in the second and third decades.
- Age is common in the second and third decades.
- M÷ F= 2÷1.
- It accounts for 2% of all chondromas.

Location

- Proximal humerus (at least 50%), and are the most common sites.

Signs

- They often present due to swelling due to the superficiality of the lesion.
- Pain may be due to stimulation of adjacent tendons.

Imaging

- Small soft tissue mass 2 to 3 cm (with calcification in 50% of cases).
- It is often the major component of a radiolucent tumor.
- Saucerization is seen with the thickening of the compensatory cortex.
- It does not extend into the modular canal.
- HighT2 on MRI.
- Rarely covers all of the main bone.

The Potential for Malignancy

- It is benign. It rarely becomes chondrosarcoma.

Macroscopic Pathology

- Varies from 1 to 5 cm.
- A cartilaginous mass is a lobule that is covered with fibrous tissue with a raised periosteum.
- The lower cortex is smoothly excavated.
- It is separated from the medullary space by a thin layer of cortical bone.

Microscopic Pathology

- It is more cellular than endochromes.
- Has a mild nuclear atypia.

Treatment

- Marginal resection involving the lower cortex.

Other

- It is connected to the insertion site of the tendon and ligament

DD

- Periosteal osteosarcoma: It is more likely to be diaphyseal and has a periosteal reaction with sunburst or hair-on-end.
- Periosteal Chondrosarcoma (Juxtacort Cialis: Patients older, and the lesion size is larger) 4 to 5 cm. None of the periosteal chondrosarcomas was less than 3 cm.
- Osteochondroma: The cortex and bone marrow cavity are associated with the tumor, unlike periosteal chondroma.
- Osteomyelitis: Has symptoms of infection and lacks a large soft tissue component.

(FCT & NOF) Fibrous Xanthoma

Included

- Fibrous Cortical Defect (FCT)
- Non-ossifying Fibroma (NOF)

Demographics

- FCD is the most common bone lesion in 30% of the normal population in the first 2 decades of life before closure.
- Peak age of both: It is the second decade.
- Rarely seen on radiographs after age 20.
- M ÷ F = 2 ÷ 1.

Source

- The difference between FCD and NOF is in the original size and location. The size of the cortical defect fibrosis is smaller, usually less than three centimeters.
- By forming reactive bone from the environment, improvement is created.
- May be due to edema and bleeding at the site of the ligament/tendon growth plate.

Location

- In metaphyses, long bones are usually seen on the posterior side of the medial.
- The distal femoral proximal tibia and distal tibia are the most common sites of involvement, respectively.
- With age: go from metaphysics to diaphysis. Most cases improve with age. Rarely, the tumor increases in size and leads to pathological fractures.

- 55% is around the knees.
- It is generally rare in the upper extremities, but proximal humerus and then distal radius are more common.
- It is sometimes multifocal and involves more or less symmetrically several metaphysical regions.
- Can rarely involve the diaphysis.

Clinical Signs

- FCD is asthmatic.
- NOF is asthmatic except for large lesions in which:
  - Pain, focal bone enlargement, and pathological fractures may occur.
- The risk of fracture is higher in the following cases:
  - It is larger than three centimeters.
  - More than half the transverse diameter of the bone is involved.
  - Weight-bearing is seen in the bone.
  - Distal tibial lesion.

Imaging

- The FCD is smaller and centered in the cortex. A size less than or equal to 3cm is suggested for the FCD. Although not everyone agrees.
- NOF is up to 7 cm or larger. Lucent margin is eccentric. It is located in the metaphyseal modular canal of the long bones. It does not usually break the cortex but has a slight thinning or scalloping bulge. The pod is like a bunch of grapes.
- Both have thin sclerotic rims.
- Do not have mineralization inside the lesion.
- Both lesions often resolve spontaneously in late adolescence. It improves from the environment to the center and begins to sclerosis.

MRI

- Isointense to muscle: T1.
- The variable T2 usually has a low signal due to its fibrosis content. In the presence of cystic areas, which are also common, a signal increase is seen in T 2.
- The surrounding bone is normal (no edema).
- The surrounding rim has a low signal at T 2.

BS

Routine is not done. The following may be seen if:

- Moderate uptake: When the lesion is healing.
- No activity: The lesion has healed.
- Severe uptake: In fracture.

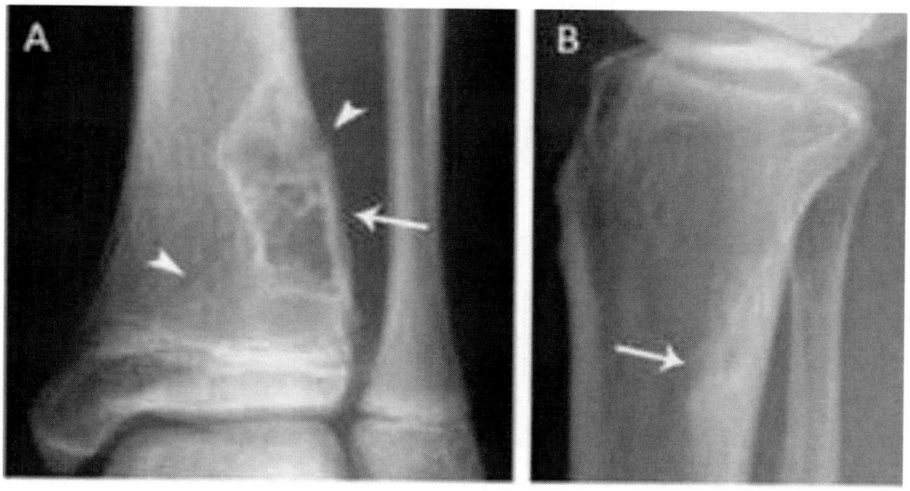

Figure 2-9. NOF of distal tibia with pathologic fracture (left). Healed NOF of proximal tibia (right).

Macroscopic Pathology

- Tan, brown or yellow.
- Extensive cystic changes, bleeding, or necrosis can occur, especially in large lesions.

Microscopic Pathology

- Is a fibrohistocytic proliferation.
- Spindle cell bundles (fibroblasts) have a tornado pattern.
- Multinucleated giant cells are seen. The margins of these cells are angular and have pycnotic nuclei.
- Histiocytes are phage in areas of fat lesions. A large number of these cells give a macroscopic yellow appearance to the contents of the lesion during surgery.
- The homozygous pigment may be seen, which, if present in large amounts, is responsible for the brown-tan appearance of the contents of the lesion during surgery.

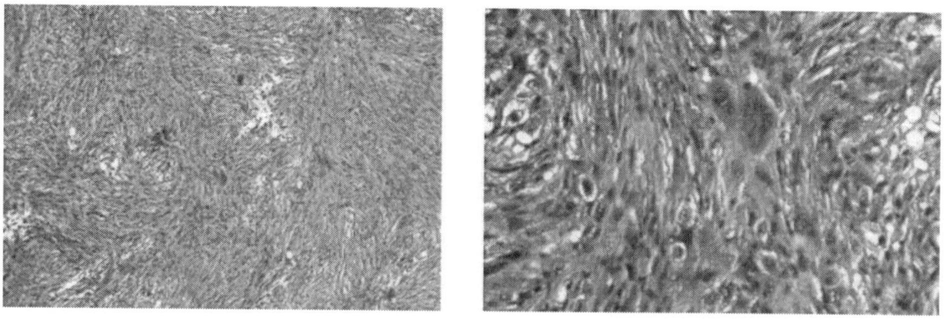

Figure 2-10. Non-Ossifying fibroma: Storiform pattern of fibroblasts with scattered benign giant cells, foamy histiocyte.

Treatment

- If you are at risk for a pathological fracture, enlarge your bone, or have a secondary ABC: Curettage and bone grafting are recommended.

- If it is broken, conservative treatment is performed until the fracture heals, and then curettage is performed with or without a bone graft.
- It is the most common site of pathological fracture in the distal tibia, although the most common site is the distal femoral tumor. Therefore, there is a greater tendency to perform surgery on distal tibial tumors.

Other

- It should not appear in adults for the first time. It usually improves at this age and has an opaque appearance.
- The presence of a soft tissue mass outside the tumor denies the diagnosis of FCD or NOF.
- In thin bones such as fibula or ulna, it can fill the entire canal because, with growth and shortening, the lesion extends from one cortex to the opposite cortex. In these places with UBC, ABC, LCH has a differential diagnosis.
- Associated with vitamin D-resistant rickets and osteomalacia. After removing the tumor, the above diseases disappear.
- 8% of NOF is multiple:
    - Familial or associated with neurofibromatosis or Campanachi's syndrome.
    - Multiple lesions, especially in the metaphyseal region, can stick together and increase the risk of pathological fractures by creating a large lesion.

DD

- Cortical desmoid: Located in the posterior femoral distal medial. The external cortex is sunken. In contrast, the external cortex is prominent in NOF. Its margin is less clear. Sclerosis surrounds and swells soft tissue.
- FD: It is central, diaphyseal or metadiaphysical.
- Abscess: In MRI, the edema has soft tissue and bone marrow. Its T2 high component is larger.
- Osteoid Osteoma Sclerosis is more pronounced. Edema has more soft tissue and bone marrow, its clinical symptoms are specific.
- ABC :It is more widespread. Multiple fluid levels in MRI are its diagnostic feature.
- UBC: It is central.

Cortical Desmoid

Other Names

- Peristaltic desmoid

Definition

- Reactive lesion in the posterior metaphysis of the distal femur in adolescents.

Creation Mechanism

- Magnus adductor muscle is created by stretching.

Epidemiology

- Common between the ages of 10 and 15.

Clinical Signs

- The pain

Imaging

- Facial radiographs rotated 20 to 45 degrees outward to help locate the lesion.
- Cortical erosion with sclerosis is seen in the posterior metaphyseal of the distal femur.

MRI

- Seen in dark at T1 and light at T2.
- Severe edema around T2 is clearly seen around the lesion.

Bone Scan

- Increases absorption.

Fibrous dysplasia
Another name: Lichtenstein- Jaffe disease

Epidemiology

- 5% includes all benign bone tumors.
- The monostatic type is 8 to 10 times more common than the most common poly osteotic type.
- 70% of patients are under 30 years old and 30% are over 30 years old.
- The type of polyesthetic is seen at a younger age.
- M = F.

Definition

- Dysplastic anomaly of ossicular mesenchymal tissue.
- Inability of the Lamar bone to be made by the skeletal tissue due to the cessation of the process of converting the woven bone to the Lamar.
- This condition can be local or diffuse, and based on this, the disease is divided into two types: monostotic and polyostotic.

Location

- In the monostatic type, the most common site of involvement is craniofacial, followed by ribs.
- The monomial type usually involves the unilateral lower extremity and the pelvis on the same side.

Clinical Signs

- Monosteotomy is an accidental finding. Swelling or deformity is the most common symptom if it is symptomatic.
- In general, the size of the lesion, the likelihood of clinical symptoms, and the extent and severity of skeletal involvement in polyosteopathy are more severe, and the age of onset of symptoms is lower.
- Pain, tenderness and lameness may also be present.
- Patients with pathological fractures, especially in the long bones, may present as primary symptoms.
- Bowing, LLD, craniofacial deformity, scoliosis are other symptoms.
- Usually during puberty, the growth of the lesion reaches a stable state.
- The most common extra-skeletal symptom is coffee milk spots on the skin.
- Coffee milk stains can match the location of bone lesions.
- The most common endocrine disorder is premature puberty in women.
- Other endocrine disorders include acromegaly, Cushing's disease, hyperparathyroidism, and hyperthyroidism.
- McCune-Albright syndrome includes the following triad
    - Polyesthetic Osteopathy FD.
    - Skin pigmentation (Café au lait) is in the form of coast of main.
    - Premature puberty or other endocrine disorders.
    - Complete triad is uncommon, two out of three are sufficient for diagnosis.
    - F> M is especially more common in women than men.
    - Leontiasis tissue ossea (lion face): Polyesthetic osteoporosis FD, with craniofacial involvement. It is rare.
    - Mazabraud syndrome: Very rare. FD mostly polyesthetic (with mix and intramuscular).

- Hypophosphatemic and osteomalacic rickets can be associated with mono and polyosteopic type. It may improve with FD treatment.

Imaging

- Clear border, ground glass view.
- Long bone, rib, pelvic diaphysis are most often involved.
- Marginal sclerosis with variable thickness is seen.
- Endosteal congestion is sometimes seen.
- There are some cases of chondroid calcification.
- The periosteal reaction can only be seen if it breaks or becomes malignant.
- Long lesion in a long bone.
- Shepherd's crook Deformity: The varicose veins of the neck and proximal to the femoral shaft. It is created by repetitive micro-structures.
- Parrot beak deformity: Stress fracture along the medial femoral neck in this disease. The radiolucent line is seen perpendicular to the femoral cortex. Surrounded by reactive bone.
- Bowing coxa vera, and protoblast acetabulum can also be seen.
- Spine: A lesion with a definite margin, leucent, dilated with multiple.
- Septations, usually seen in the vertebral body. Sometimes found in posterior elements. Rarely associated with collapse or deviation of the spine and compression of the spinal cord.

CT

- Used for FD in pelvis, spine, skull.
- Suitable for showing lack of periosteal reaction.

MRI

Low à intermediate: T1.

Low àhigh: T2.

Low signal frame with variable thickness can be seen in both views, which indicates sclerosis around the lesion.

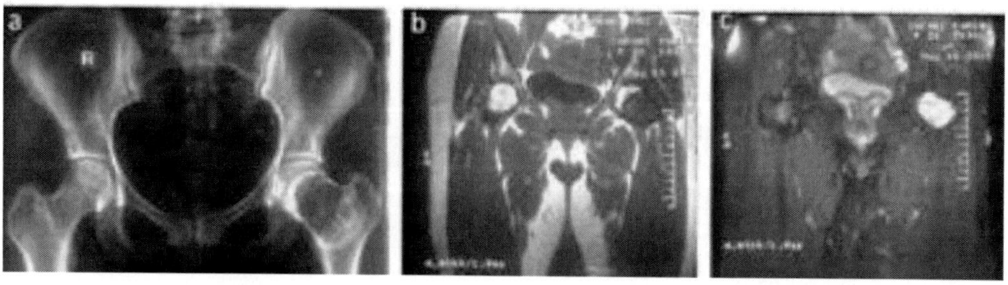

Figure 2-11. Fibrous dysplasia in left femoral neck.

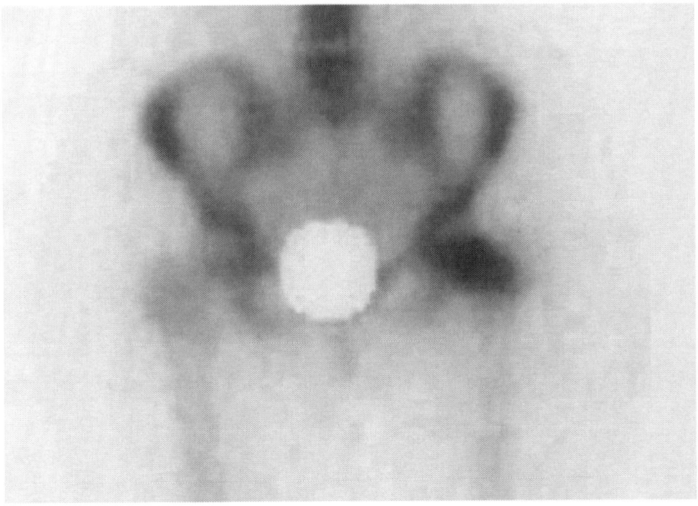

Figure 2-12. Increase in uptake in left femoral neck in bone scan.

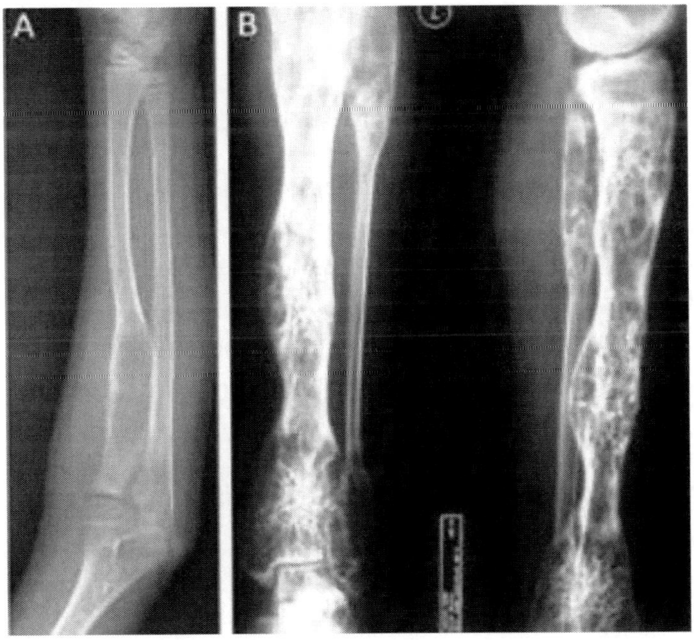

Figure 2-13. Mono osteotic Fibrous dysplasia in radius (left) Polyosteotic fibrous dysplasia in tibia and fibula (right).

BS

- It is useful for diagnosing the type of osteotic osteoporosis.
- Has normal activity or increased absorption.

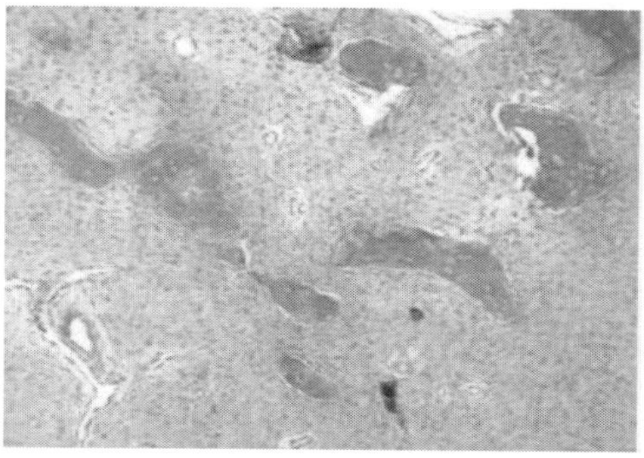

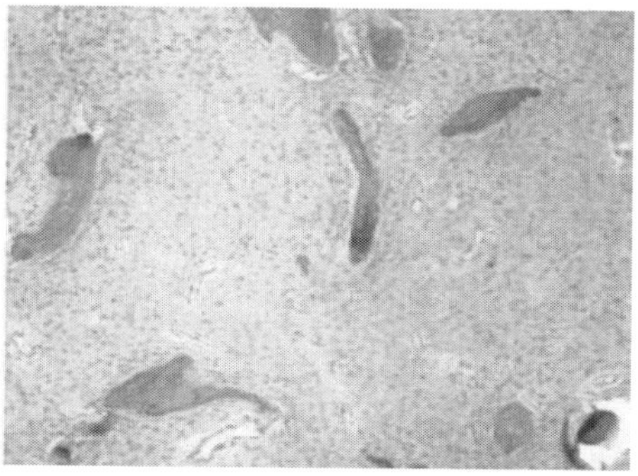

Figure 2-14. Fibrous dysplasia: Branching and anastomosing irregular trabecula of woven bone with no osteoblastic rimming in fibrous stroma.

Malignant Potential

- Rarely malignant.
- It can be present in both mono and polyesthetic types.
- It can occur with or without a history of radiotherapy.
- Pain and swelling with rapid onset, destruction of the cortex, and the presence of soft tissue masses are symptoms of malignancy.
- It becomes MFH of fibrosarcoma, chondrosarcoma, or osteosarcoma.

Treatment

- Usually conservative.
- Both mono and polyostotic types decline or stop growing at puberty, but the deformities that develop remain.
- Bisphosphonates are prescribed to relieve symptoms in the polyesthetic type.

Surgery Is Recommended in the Following Cases

1) Fracture
2) Deformity
3) Symptomatic lesion
4) Compression of the nerves

Other

- Fibrosis dysplasia is the most common benign rib lesion.
- During menstruation or pregnancy, it can be painful due to the presence of an estrogen receptor inside the tumor.

The Enlargement of the Lesion Can Be due to Three Reasons

- Becoming malignant
- Cystic degeneration
- Secondary ABC

DD

Monoaesthetic

- SBC: It is more lucent, it is more expansile, it moves away from the growth plate with age.
- ABC: It is eccentric inside the bone, it clearly thins the cortex; there is fluid level.
- GCT: It is eccentric inside the bone, centered at the junction of the metaphyseal epiphysis. It is more likely to go to the subchondral bone.
- NOF: It is eccentric, located inside the bone, in the metaphysis. It heals from the environment to the center. There is no ossification inside the lesion.
- Osteo fibrous dysplasia OFD: Always located in the TIA or fibula, located in the anterior cortex.
- Intramedullary Osteosarcoma: It has a permeative margin, mineralzation is seen with more density, the appearance of the lesion changes over time, if it is thicker.
- Paget disease (lytic phase): Older, thicker cortex and trabeculae, increased Alp.
- Liposclerosing myxofibrous tumor of bone: seen only in the intertrochanter region of the femur and is brighter in T2. Contains fat speckles.

DD

Polyesthetic

- Multiple enchondroma: can spread to the epiphysis. Radiolucent lines extend from the growth plate into the metaphysis (fluted - column sign).
- Neuro Fibromatosis: Long bone deformity without density changes in FD.
- Multiple NOFs: There are multiple NOFs with non-skeletal changes. It is also called jaffe campanacci syndrome.

Shepherd's Staff Deformity Can Be Seen in the Following Cases

- FD
- Paget's disease
- Osteogenesis imperfecta

OSTEO FIBROUS DYSPLASIA (O.F.D)

- Other names: Ossifying fibroma in fibula and tibia, Campanacci syndrome or Juvenile adamantinoma.

Definition

- Benign fibroosseous lesion is usually in the anterior cortex of the midbrain in children or infants.

Epidemiology

- It is rare.
- It is usually seen in the first two decades of life. It may also be seen at birth. Two-thirds of cases are diagnosed under the age of five.
- Both sexes are equally involved.

Location

- TIA (78 to 80%) is more commonly seen in the proximal or lower 1.3.
- It can be bilateral, it can involve the fibula on either side or the other side.
- Unilateral tibial and fibula involvement is typical.
- All cases reported were seen in TIA, fibula or both. In cases of fibula involvement alone, it is usually seen in the lower third.

Clinical Signs

- May be asymptomatic
- Local pain or swelling
- Anterior bowing
- Pathological fractures

Imaging

- Lucent lesion, multicellular, marked sclerotic margin, 10% likely to involve medullary canal. Multiple lesions next to each other give the tibia a bubble tooth appearance.
- The length of the lesion varies from 3 cm to the involvement of the entire bone.
- Anterior and lateral tibial curvature is present in more than 80% of cases.
- Pathological fractures and even pseudoarthritis have been reported.

CT

Indicates a lack of rupture of the cortex within the surrounding soft tissue.

MRI

Low to intermediate signal: T1

High signal: T2

The above lesions are isolated with areas of the normal cortex, which have a low signal in T1 and T2.

BS

Increases absorption

Potential for malignancy:

- Probably does not exist.
- Slow growth in the child until the age of 15, then self-improvement or regression.
- Can be locally aggressive and commonly causes local recurrence.

Potential for Malignancy

- Probably does not exist.
- Slow growth in the child until the age of 15, then self-improvement or regression.
- Can be locally aggressive and commonly causes local recurrence.

Microscopic Pathology

- In the form of loose bundles composed of fibroblast-like cells with a round inflatable appearance.
- The central region of the tumor is predominantly fibrous and may have undergone micizomatous changes.

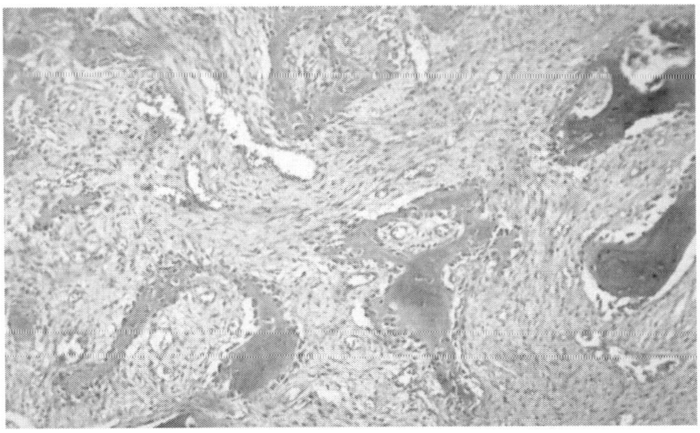

Figure 2-15. Osteo fibrous dysplasia: Woven bone trabecula with prominent osteoblastic rimming and Spindle cell proliferation without atypia.

Treatment

- Surgery for children if they have one or more of the following:
  - Pseudoarthritis.
  - Severe curvature.
  - Large lesion at risk of Fx or broken
- Types of surgeries
  - Curettage + Cryo + Bone Graft.
  - Extensive bone resection and graft

Other

- The relationship with adamantinoma is discussed.
- In fibula, because it is small, it can take up all the thickness of the bone.

- 2/3 occurs before the age of 5.
- It may even be seen in infants.
- Some authors believe that treatment is conservative even in pathological fractures. Accordingly, if the surgeon intends to correct the deformity, it is better to wait until puberty because surgery is associated with a high recurrence at a young age.

DD

- Adamantinoma: Older age, larger lesion, and more aggressive.
- FD: In the centralized canal medulla, the cortex is thin but has no bubbly appearance.
- OM: Severe soft tissue edema and bone marrow. Different clinical symptoms.
- Single lesions (individual lesions) have the appearance of frosted glass, but their accumulation together gives the bone a bubble or sawtooth appearance.

DESMOPLASTIC FIBROMA (DF)

Other names: Bone desmoid tumor

Definition

- It is a single locally aggressive mass composed of myofibroblasts with abundant collagen deposition.

Epidemiology

- Very rare: It accounts for 1% of primary bone tumors.
- Soft tissue is 5-15 times less common than desmoid tumor.
- It is more common in adolescents and young adults. It is more common in the second and third decades.
- M = F.

Source

- Intramuscular type of desmoid is soft tissue.

Location

- The most common sites involved are long bones, including the femur, tibia, humerus, and radius.
- Other areas involved include the skull, mandible, pelvis, and spine.

- In some references, the most common site involved is the craniofacial bones.
- The most specific area involved is the mandibular area of the mandible.
- It is usually metaphysical. It can also affect the epiphysis.

Clinical Signs

- It is asymptomatic until it grows.
- Chronic pain or swelling are the most common symptoms.
- Pathological fractures and deformities can be the primary symptoms.
- Pathological fractures are seen in 15%.

Imaging

- Tibial, geographic, bone dilator and leucent. It has a definite margin and thin sclerotic rim is commonly seen around it.
- The zone of transition is narrow.
- Destruction of the cortex and invasion of the surrounding soft tissue are often seen.
- Due to trabeculae inside the lesion, it has a soapy or honeycomb floor appearance.
- MRI:
  - Low signal: T 1.
  - Low signal: T 2.
  - A low signal at T2 indicates sclerosis or collagen.

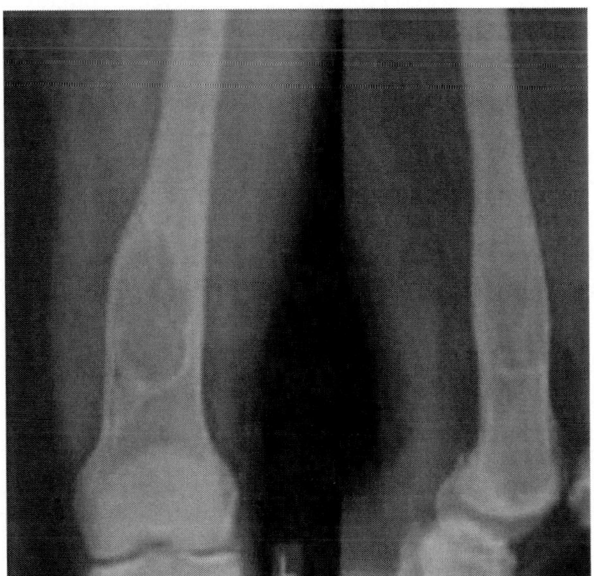

Figure 2-16. Desmoplastic fibroma in the distal femoral metaphysis.

BS

- Increased absorption

Malignant Potential

- Locally aggressive and slow-growing.
- Local recurrence is 72% with curettage and 16% following resection. Some studies have reported a local recurrence of 40% with curettage.
- Local recurrence is seen up to 8 years later.

Macroscopic Pathology

- Typical size is 3 to 10 cm. Up to 20 cm has also been seen.
- It has a white-gray color with a fibrous and firm consistency.

Microscopic Pathology

- Spindle-shaped fibroblasts within the abundant and dense collagen matrix.
- The pathology is similar to soft tissue fibromatosis.
- It is hypocellular and mitosis is slightly observed.

Treatment

- The preferred treatment for most authors is wide resection. Recurrence has also been seen with this method.
- Simple curettage and bone grafting have a 40% recurrence.
- Extensive curettage may be an acceptable treatment. This method maintains better performance than resection.
- Adjuvant treatments used in soft tissue desmoid tumors (radiotherapy, anti-inflammatory drugs, tamoxifen, and cytotoxic drugs) may play a therapeutic role, but there is little supporting evidence.
- Does not metastasize.

Other

- Eating bone cortex should not be confused with malignancy. It is seen in 29% of cases.
- May be associated with fibrous dysplasia and melorheostosis.

DD

- GCT: Both can spread to the epiphysis. GCT is round and desmoplastic fibroma is oval.
- Fibrous dysplasia: covers a longer segment of bone, has a ground glass appearance, the sclerotic rim is often seen.
- ABC: It is more central inside the bone and has a dilated view, not the spindle view common in desmoplastic fibroids.
- NOF: Inside the bone is eccentric with a margin of lobules. Rim has sclerosis.
- SBC: It looks like a desmoplastic fibroma on radiography, but on the contrary, it is clear on T2. It has a liquid appearance on MRI and CT.
- Low-grade fibrosarcoma: has permeative growth, the zone of transition is wider.

- Low-grade osteosarcoma with fibroblasts predominance: It has a mineralized matrix although they are similar in histology.

Simple Bone Cyst

Other names:
Unicameral bone cyst, solitary bone cyst

Epidemiology

- 85% are seen in less than 20 years. The age peak is four to ten years.
- It is twice as common in males as in females.
- 3% of all biopsy neoplasms of the bone.

Source

- A cavity is a chamber lined with mesothelial cells. It contains serous fluid or serosangin.
- It may be due to a local defect in metaphyseal remodeling due to impaired interstitial fluid drainage, leading to necrosis and cyst formation.
- Cyst fluid contains prostaglandins, oxygen-free radicals, interleukins, cytokines, and metalloproteins, all of which may be involved in bone resorption.

Location

- Can be seen on any bone.
- It is located in the long bones in the central area of the metaphysis.
- Can migrate into the diaphysis with age.
- 90% are found in the proximal humerus, proximal femur, and proximal TIA. Fifty percent is found alone in Homer.
- Over the age of 20, ilium, calcaneus, and talus are the most common areas of conflict.

Clinical Signs

- Most are asymptomatic.
- Rarely have pain and swelling.
- In more than 50% of cases (two-thirds of cases) occur with pathological fractures.
- Broad bones are rarely broken and are asymptomatic.
- Lesions usually heal spontaneously with age.

Imaging

- Lucent.
- Geographic, with defined margins.
- Central metadiaphysis.
- Bone expansion is negligible.
- Never pierce the cortex.
- Prominent bony blades inside the cyst may give it the appearance of several cavities. This condition is seen after the healing of pathological fractures in the field of simple bone cysts.
- Expands to the pharynx.
- The margins are smooth and have no sclerotic rim.
- Matrix mineralization or soft tissue expansion.
- Unlike ABC, the width of the lesion does not exceed the adjacent growth plate.
- Has no positive reaction unless broken.
- Fallen fragment sign: A broken piece falls from the bone cortex into the dependent area. The diagnostic sign of a simple bone cyst is a fracture. It is seen in 20% of cases and is a sign that the cyst is empty.
- Trap door sign. The broken piece remains attached to the periosteum but bends into the cyst.
- Rising bubble sign is the appearance of air bubbles inside the bone at the highest part of the cyst. This condition can be seen on a CT scan or plain radiograph after a fracture and is characteristic of a simple bone cyst.
- Pathological fractures can lead to stunted growth or osteonecrosis of the femoral head.

CT

- Can show a fluid-fluid level. This condition occurs following a fracture.

MRI

- It usually has a liquid signal.
- It can have a fluid-fluid level.
- Low: intermediate T1.
- Heterogenous high T2.
- Increases environmental absorption with Gadolinium.
- When it breaks, it becomes fluid-level, the signal becomes heterogeneous, and the amplification of the peripheral signal becomes up to 1 cm thick.

BS

- Increased environmental absorption, without activity in the center.
- Bs may be normal.

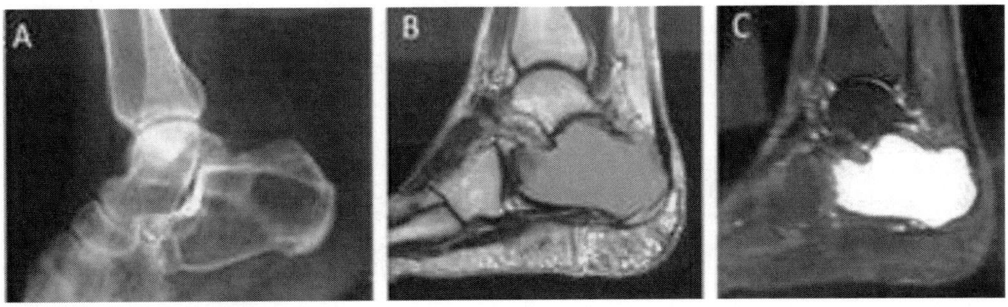

Figure 2-17. Simple bone cyst in calcaneus.

Macroscopic Pathology

- Large intra-medullary cavity of bone filled with yellow fluid with low viscosity.
- When there is a cavity, it is sometimes divided into several cavities due to bony septa.
- The single wall is a thin layer of yellow-tan fibrous tissue, usually less than 1 mm thick, filled with several bony blades.

Microscopic Pathology

- The area around the cyst is covered with a fibrous layer containing fibroblasts and lacks epithelium.
- Inflammatory filling cells of attached arteries and multinucleated giant cells are also seen.
- Hemosiderin pigment and cloud macrophages are seen focally.
- Reactive osteogenesis with overt osteoblasts is seen at the fracture site.
- Mineralized fibrin is seen inside the cyst wall as cementoid bodies.

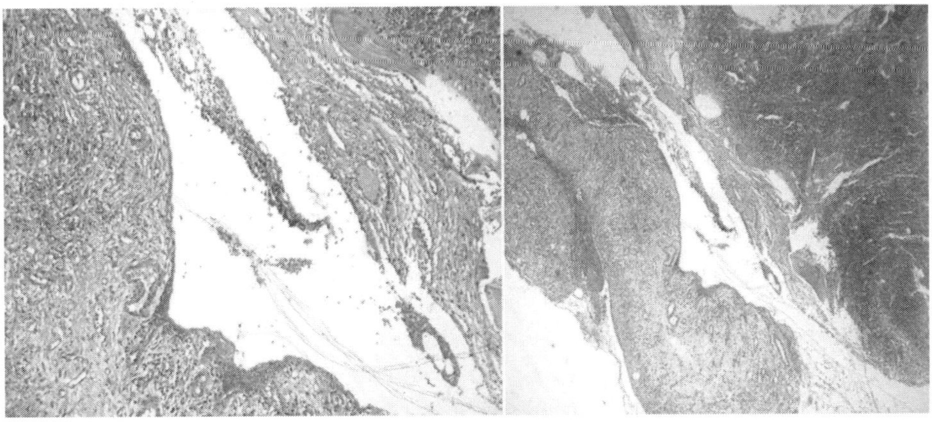

Figure 2-18. Unicameral bone cyst: The area around the cyst is covered with a fibrous layer containing fibroblasts and lacks epithelium.

Treatment

- It can regress, either spontaneously or following a fracture.
- The probability of cyst healing due to pathological fracture is very low (less than 5%).
- Small lesions in the upper limbs are followed by serial radiography.

- Large lesions (prone to pathological fractures, symptomatic lesions, and lower extremity lesions are usually treated by curettage with or without bone grafts, or by aspiration and injection of steroids, bone marrow, or demineralized bone matrix or other materials).
- In case of pathological fracture in the upper limb, conservative treatment is performed until the fracture heals, then a separate treatment system is considered.
- In case of pathological fracture in proximal femoral cysts, surgical treatment with curettage, transplantation.
- Bone and internal fixation are performed.
- Flexible nails have been used in femoral and arm fractures, thus eliminating the need for casting.
- Aspiration and double-needle steroid injection are the treatment of choice.
- If no signs of improvement are seen on the radiograph after 2 months of injection, re-injections are given. Repeated injections are successful in more than 90% of cases. Normally at least three injections should be given. It is not recommended to perform a follow-up radiography earlier than two to three months, because if it improves sooner than this time, there will be no signs of improvement on the radiograph.
- Poor prognosis for injection therapy: Multi-cavity radiograph, large cyst size, active lesion (cyst 1 cm apart), and age less than ten years.
- Bone graft curettage should be used to treat large cysts in weight-bearing bones that are prone to fractures, such as the proximal femur.
- The use of allografts or bone substitutes provides excellent healing without the discomfort of removing bone from the patient.
- Recurrence after injection or curettage and the bone graft is about 20%.

Other

- CT helps find the fallen fragment.
- Types of simple bone cysts: Active) Cysts are 1 cm apart (and inactive) Cysts are more than 1 cm away (active type tends to grow more.
- Multiple radiographic, fluoroscopic, or CT scans are needed to find a fallen fragment.

DD

- ABC: It is very dilated, it has an eccentric location inside the bone, it can have a monolayer periosteal reaction. It has liquid-liquid surfaces, and numerous cavities. The diameter of the cyst is larger than the diameter of the pharynx when it is central.
- Enchondroma: The margins are lobed. The outside of the limbs should have a cartilaginous type inside the mineralized lesion. Otherwise enchondroma is not an issue.
- Fibrous dysplasia: has a dense glass density and no bone trabeculae.
- Fallen has no fragment.
- GCT: It spreads to the subchondral bone. The phase is not open and age is high.

Extras

- Dependent fluid: A heavier fluid that settles inside the cyst. At T2, the signal is lower than the lighter liquid and darker. This precipitated fluid contains blood or protein
- Liquid-fluid surfaces are seen in two cases in simple bone cysts:
  - Fracture,
  - Cyst fluid has a high protein content.

ABC

Epidemiology

- M = F.
- Most often seen in 5 to 20 years. 80% are seen under 20 years. The peak age is in the second decade.
- % 1 constitutes all primary biopsy tumors.
- Source
  - It may be due to a venous obstruction or an arterial-venous fistula.
  - The capillaries inside the cyst are in contact with the capillaries of the general circulation, which can cause bleeding during surgery.
  - May be associated with trauma.
  - Primer is 70% of cases.
  - The secondary accounts for 30% of other tumors (benign / malignant).
- Place
  - It can affect almost all bones.
  - 20% is found in long bones. It is more common in femur, TB, and then Homer, respectively.
  - Distal femur, proximal tibia, and humerus are common sites
  - It is mostly metaphysical and eccentric in long bones.
  - It is more common in the bones of the ankle than the wrist.
  - Posterior element is usually involved in the spine. It is common in thoracic, lumbar, cervical, and sacral, respectively.

Clinical Signs

- Pain and swelling are typical symptoms.
- 10 to 20% occur with pathological fractures.
- Nerve symptoms or cord compression are seen during spinal involvement.

Imaging

- Its most obvious appearance is severe dilatation of the periosteum and a thin layer of cortex beneath it. Severely expansile.

- Lucent and Geographic.
- Multi-local.
- The rim has no sclerosis / is insignificant.
- It is eccentric, but large lesions may appear central, especially in smaller bones.
- The cortex is extremely thin. It may be intact but may not be seen on radiographs.
- Periosteal new bone can be seen in solid lesions or pathological fractures.
- It can rarely have a soft tissue component.
- In children, stunted growth or angular deformity is rarely caused by invasion of the pharynx.
- Can pass through the disc and engage an adjacent nut.

CT

- Useful for finding occult-cortex not seen on radiographs.
- Indicates internal septation and fluid-fluid level.

MRI

- Heterogenous T1, T2 with multiple fluid-fluid levels.
- High T1 = Dependent fluid due to methemoglobin (see dependent fluid in UBC).
- Increase environmental absorption in the use of Gadolinium.

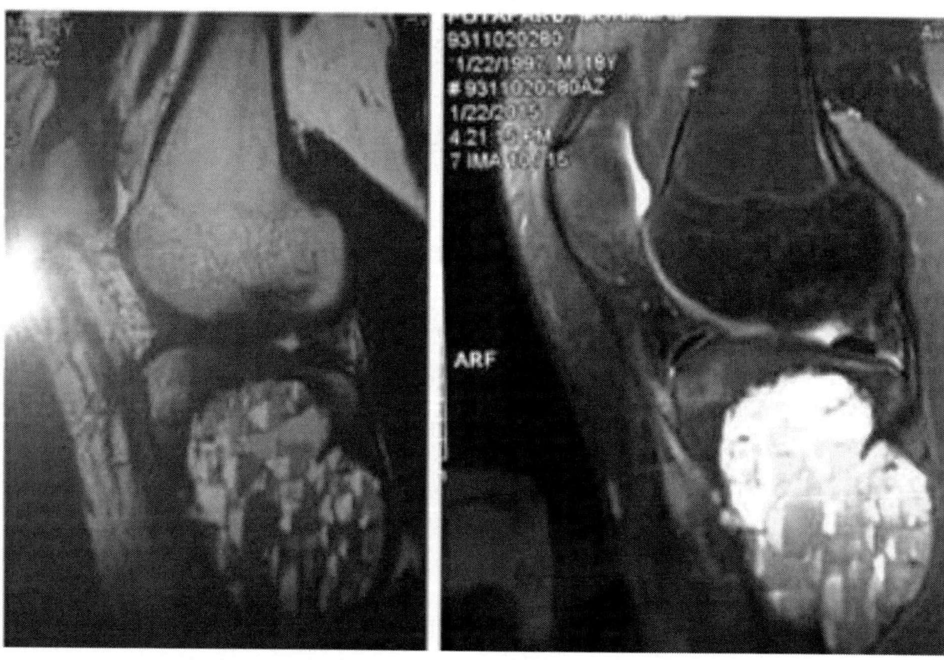

Figure 2-19. ABC in proximal tibia metaphsis.

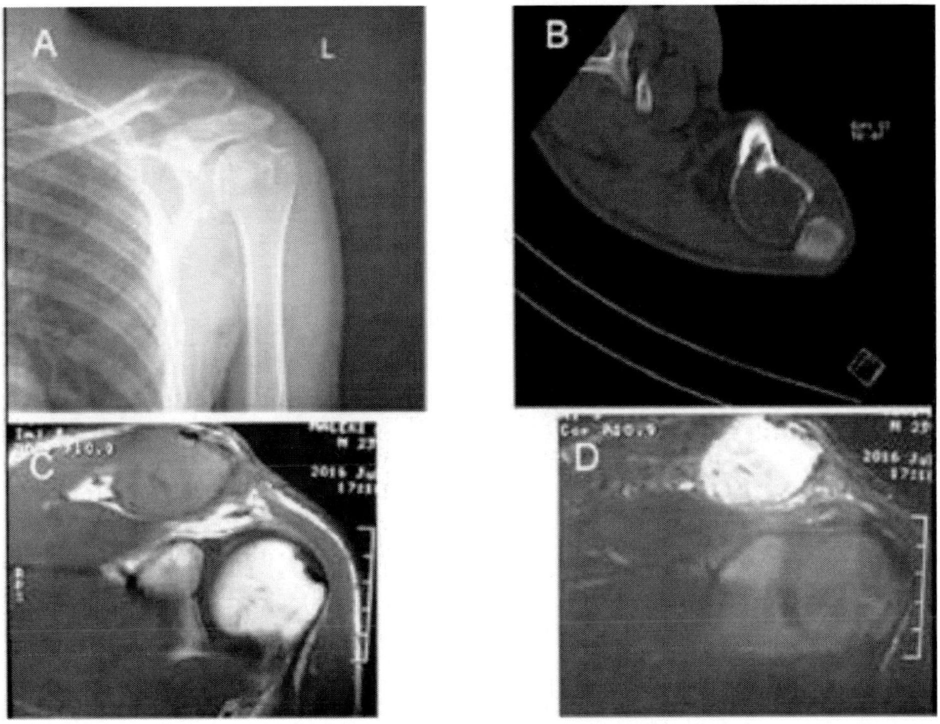

Figure 2-20. Solid ABC.

BS

- It is non-proprietary. They show peripheral activity in 64%.

The Potential for Malignancy

- Has local recurrence potential.
- Secondary ABC may be seen in sarcomas, especially osteosarcoma.
- ABC malignancy is reported to be malignant.

Macroscopic Pathology

- It is a cavity with bloody spaces separated by bony septa.
- It is limited by a thin layer of bone covered with periost.

Microscopic Pathology

- Tissue is bleeding with cave-shaped cavities separated by cellular stroma.
- Cave cavities include compressed fibroblasts and histiocytes.
- Macrophages containing hemosiderin, chronic inflammatory cells, and multinucleated giant cells are also present.
- A solid type of bone aneurysm cyst known as giant cell reparative granuloma has also been described.

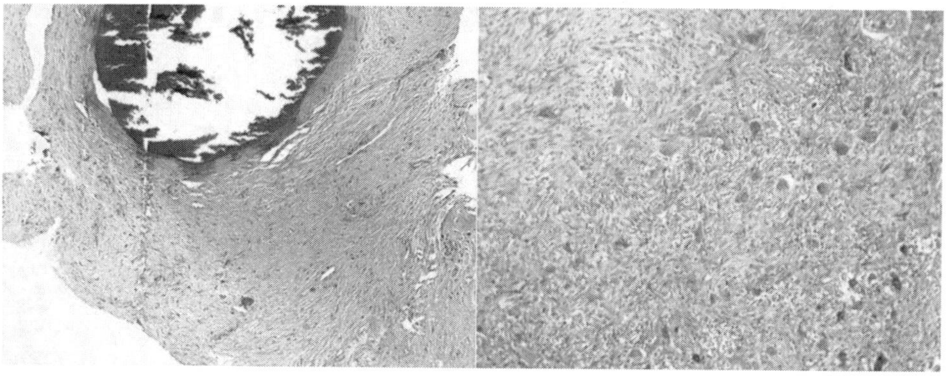

Figure 2-21. ABC: Cave cavities include compressed fibroblasts and histiocytes, Macrophages containing hemosiderin, chronic inflammatory cells, and multinucleated giant cells are also present.

Treatment

- They cause severe deformity and severe dysfunction by causing local damage.
- Spontaneous recovery (spontaneous regression) is rarely seen.
- Most untreated lesions progress.
- Complete excision of the lesion is the most effective treatment, but may be associated with severe dysfunction. In dilated bones, treatment is optional.
- Therefore, most cysts are treated with extensive curettage and bone grafting.
- It is recommended to use a tourniquet because of the possibility of bleeding during the operation.
- Recurrence is seen in 10 to 20% of cases after curettage. Recurrence is common in the first 2 years. Recurrence typically occurs in the first 6 months. Risk factors for recurrence include:
  - Age less than 15 years.
  - Centrally located cysts
- In general, 90% of patients have satisfactory long-term treatment results.
- Prolonged injection of oscalcitonin, methylprednisolone, and sclerosing agents such as Ethibloc improves the lesion.
- Arterial embolization is used in the following cases:
  - Pelvic and spinal injuries to reduce the risk of bleeding before surgery.
  - Definitive treatment in areas where curettage is difficult.
- Low-dose radiotherapy, which is associated with rapid ossification of the lesion, is recommended in the following cases Becomes:
  - Incompletely resectable.
  - Be recurrent or aggressive.
  - To prevent damage to important areas such as the spinal cord due to surgery.

Other

- Giant cell reparative granuloma in the peripheral skeleton is a solid form of ABC and is associated with USP6 rearrangement. Giant cell reparative granuloma in primary or secondary hyperparathyroidism can be seen as reactive and not tumorous.
- GCT patients are slightly older than ABCs.

- DD Lytic lesion with Fluid level:
  - SBC with fracture
  - ABC
  - GCT
  - Chondroblastoma - located in the epiphysis
  - Osteoblastoma
  - Telangiectatic osteosarcoma

Differential Diagnosis

- GCT: Less expansile. It spreads to the subchondral bone. It has solid components. No periosteal reaction. They are older.
- SBC: Central, but ABC is off-center. Its expansion is negligible, and it is a hole. The periosteal reaction occurs only when fractured. Fallen fragment view and gas bubble view are diagnostic for SBC.
- NOF: Like ABC, it has no fluid levels. It does not expand bones, except to a very small extent.
- Pseudotumor in hemophilia: Has a history of hemophilia.

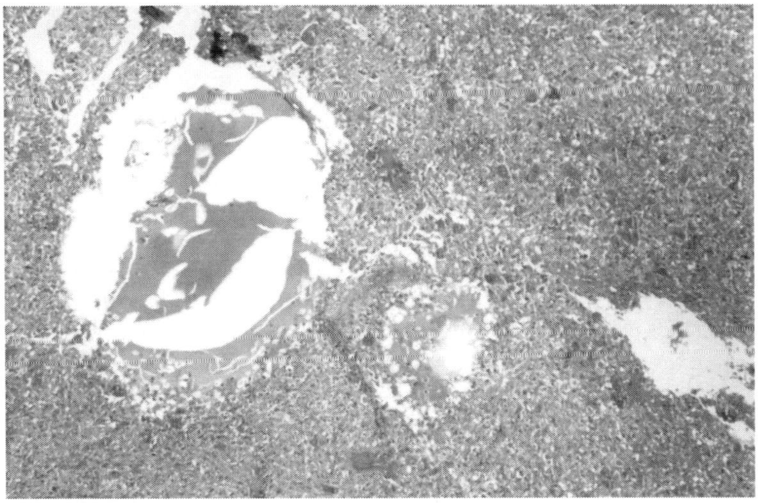

Figure 2-22. Giant cell tumor with ABC.

Secondary ABC in Benign Lesions

- Brown tumor
- GCT
- Chondroblastoma
- CMF
- LCH
- FD
- Hemangioma
- NOF
- Osteoblastoma

- SBC
- Giant cell reparative granuloma

Secondary ABC in Malignant Lesions

- Angiosarcoma
- Chondrosarcoma
- MFH
- Telangiectatic Osteosarcoma
- Hemangioendothelioma

Bone Lipoma

Other names
Intraosseous lipoma ‹Parosteal lipoma

Epidemiology

- Decades 2-8
- M ÷ F = 1.6
- 1% contains all primary bone tumors

Source

- Neoplasms of benign adult adipocytes.
- Some believe that intraosseous lipoma is a bone infarct.
- The parosteal type rises from the surface of the bone.

Location

- The modular canal is usually involved. Rarely found inside the cortex or on the surface of the bone.
- Proximal femur, calcaneus, illium, and vitia are common sites of involvement.
- The type of parosteal is seen along the diaphysis. It was formerly known as the periosteal.

Clinical Signs

- It is usually incidental.
- Achy pain can be due to intraosseous ischemia and increased pressure in that area.

- Pathological fractures are rare.
- The parosteal type can cause nerve compression or bulging (rarely).

Imaging

- Geographically, Lucent with ZOT fringe has thin, narrow or broad scleral rim.
- Calcification inside the ring-like or central lesion is seen in 57% of cases.
- The above case is pathognomic lipoma in the body of calcaneus.

Milgram Staging

- Stage 1 Cells containing viable fat only: Radiolucent with a definite margin.
- Stage 2 partial fat necrosis: calcification or ossification (central or peripheral).
- Stage 3 fat necrosis + calcification and cyst formation and proliferation of fibrosis.
- Pathognomonic view of bull's eye: In the middle of cystic degeneration, then around the fat and farthest out of the rim ossification is seen on radiography.

CT

- Fat density is the diagnostic criterion. Its Hansfield number is -60 to -100.
- Compared to BM, it may be more leukocyte due to lack of cellular elements.
- May have fluid in the center. It may have calcification in the environment or in the center.

MRI

- Isotone is a subcutaneous fat. In the T2 view, fat is suppressed and disappears with fat suppressor like the fat under the skin of the comma. Note Figure 2-18.
- High T1.
- Intermediate T2.
- No Gadolinium enhancement.
- Sometimes T2 has a higher signal than bone marrow.
- It can increase the signal in T2 due to fluid due to cystic degeneration.
- Both views can have signal reduction due to calcification (signal void).

BS

- Lack of activity or moderate activity is seen.

Other

- Parosteal Lipoma: A lipophilic, exophytic radiolucent fat mass that relies on the cortex with a variable periosteal response or variable thickening of the cavitary modular cortex not along the bone modular canal (unlike osteochondroma) and is best for pre-MRI planning.

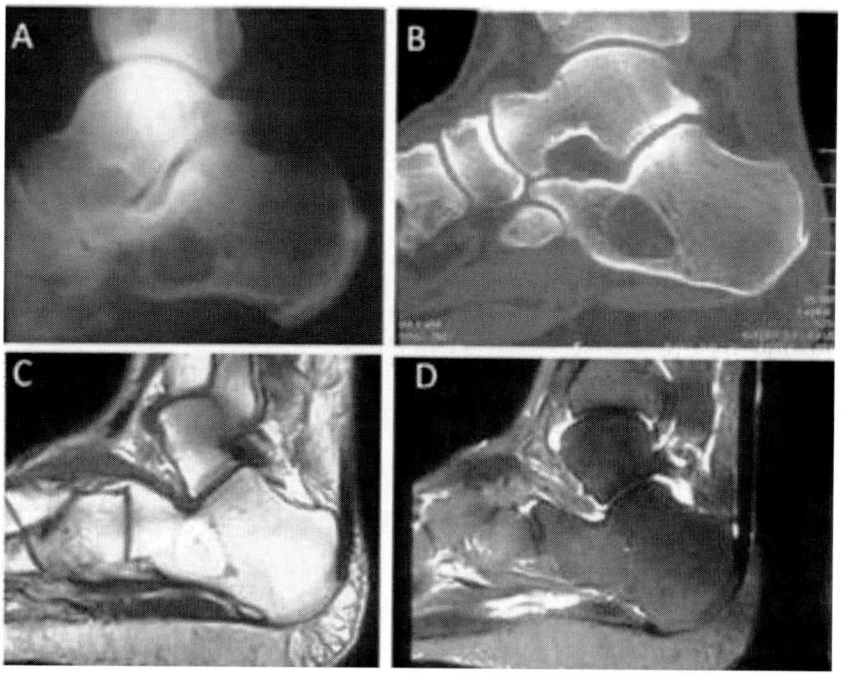

Figure 2-23. Bone lipoma: A: X-ray B: Ct scan shows intra-lipoma calcification C: MRI T1 D: MRI T2 fat-suppressed.

Macroscopic Pathology

- A lobular mass with a definite margin of adipose tissue.

Microscopic Pathology

- Contains mature adipose tissue, which is indistinguishable from soft tissue lipoma.
- Fat necrosis, and dystrophic calcification seen on radiography as opacity are common.

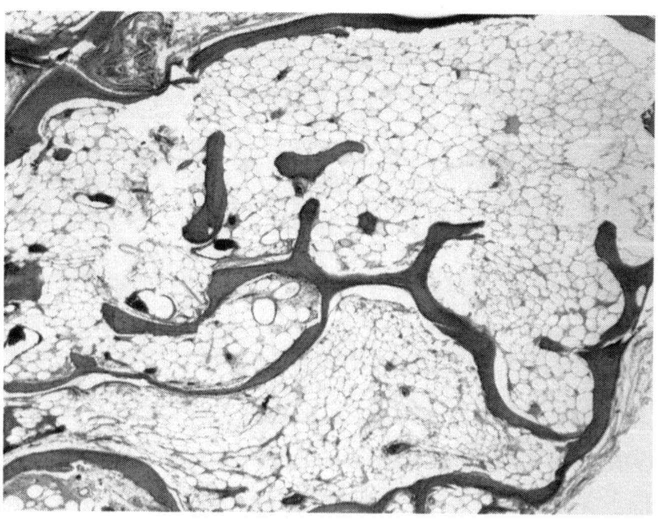

Figure 2-24. Bone lipoma: Contains mature adipose tissue.

Treatment

- Curettage + bone graft: if sympathetic.
- Excision: in the sympathetic case of the parosteal.

Malignant Posterior

- Very rare

DD

- Bone infarct: The bone does not dilate. It has a serpentine shape and a convex margin.
- SBC in calcaneus bone: No central calcification, fluid-free and fat-free. (On MRI, the signal is the opposite of lipoma)
- ABC in the calcaneus: Dilates the bone. It is more posterior and planter.
- Chondroblastoma in the calcaneus: Attached to the subtalar joint
- Pseudotumor of calcaneus: The cystic component has no central calcification
- Apart from bone infarct, other differential diagnoses were related to calcaneus lipoma.

INTRAOSSEOUS HEMANGIOMAS

Epidemiology

- It is seen in 10% of spinal autopsies.
- Mostly after the fourth decade. Incidence increases with age.
- 70% of cases are seen between 30 and 60 years
- M ÷ F = 2÷3

Source

- Most are cavernous or a mixture of capillaries and cavernous.
- A benign hamartome includes endothelial-covered spaces.

Place

- If asymptomatic cases are considered, vertebral bodies are the most common sites of involvement.
- In symptomatic cases, cranial-facial is the most common area of involvement.
- Long bones and appendicular skeleton are the next most common.
- In long bones, the tibia is the most common bone involved.

Clinical Signs

- Mostly asymptomatic.
- They can spread to the spine or cause a fracture, putting pressure on the nerve/cord.
- They may enlarge and give cord compression during pregnancy.
- Posterior element lesions are more likely to be symptomatic.

Imaging

- It is seen as a Lucent defect with a definite margin.
- In broad bones, it causes expansion. Expansion in the skull is greater in the external cortex than in the internal one.
- The vascular nature of the tumor is characterized by the appearance of a soap scab or honeycomb trabeculae.
- The upper cortex is attached and thin but not torn and does not invade soft tissue.
- The characteristic sunburst of hemangioma is seen in cranial lesions.
- The appearance of a honeycomb or polka dot or corduroy is seen due to the thickening of the vertebral trabeculae.
- Leucent lesion with a sunburst or web-like radial trabeculae spoke wheel.
- Small bones: They have a dilated appearance similar to bone aneurysmal cysts.
- Cortical and periosteal reactions can occur.

CT Scan

- Polka dot is seen in the axial cut due to thickened trabeculae.

MRI

- In hemangiomas, the limbs are dark in T1 and light in T2 due to the water content of the tumor
- In vertebral body hemangiomas, the lack of hematopoietic tissue and its replacement by the hemangioma adipose tissue causes a clear view in T1.
- Has a slight/moderate increase in contrast to Gadolinium.
- Subgroup of spinal hemangiomas in T1 view does not increase absorption: similar to metastasis (future peak type)
- The typical atypical type may damage the cortex and have a soft tissue mass.

BS

- Is variable.

The Potential for Malignancy

- Angiosarcoma is very rare.

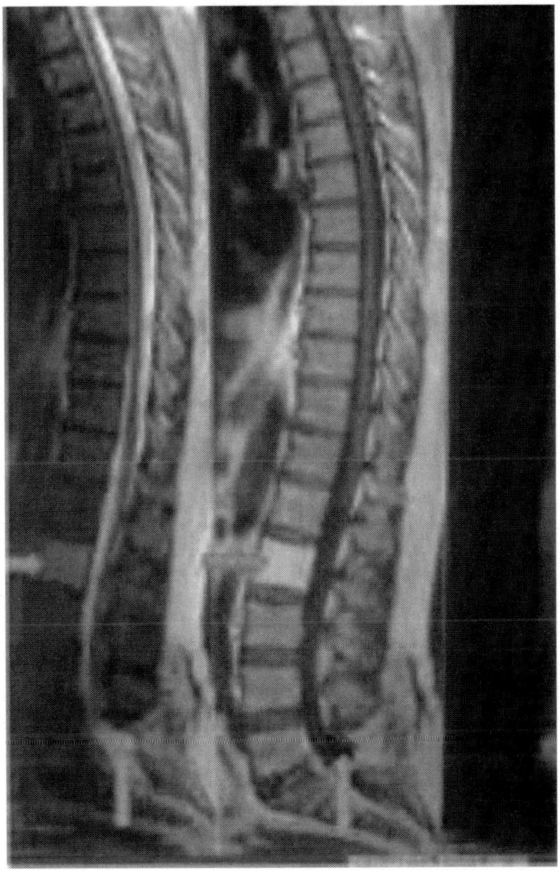

Figure 2-25. Hemangioma in L2 MRI.

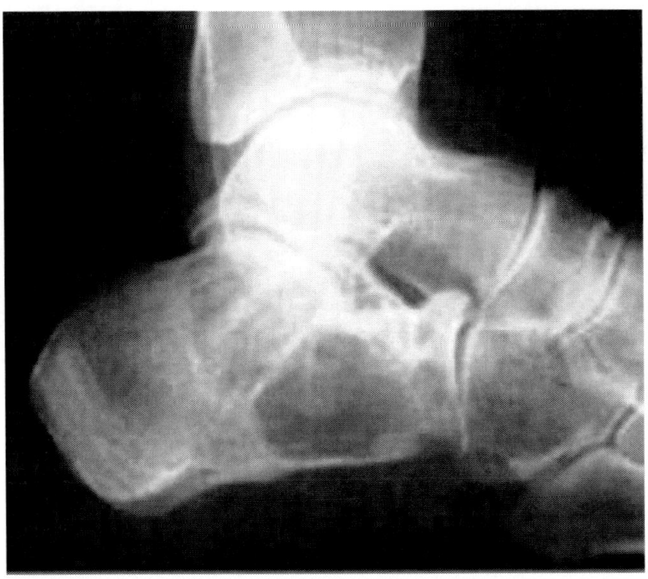

Figure 2-26. Hemangioma in calcaneus.

Macroscopic Pathology

- It is a reddish-brown or dark red medullary lesion with a definite margin.
- It is intracortical or subpriacal
- It may have the appearance of a honeycomb with sclerotic trabeculae or be boneless and have only vascular tissue.
- The peristole reaction perpendicular to the bone surface is seen in some hemangiomas.

Microscopic Pathology

- It involves the accumulation of thin-walled blood vessels.
- Cavernous arteries are more common than capillaries.
- Vascular spaces are covered with a layer of endothelial cells that can take on an epithelial appearance.
- The consul bone in the tumor area may be quite absorbed, but more commonly a number of trabeculae remain that have thickened.

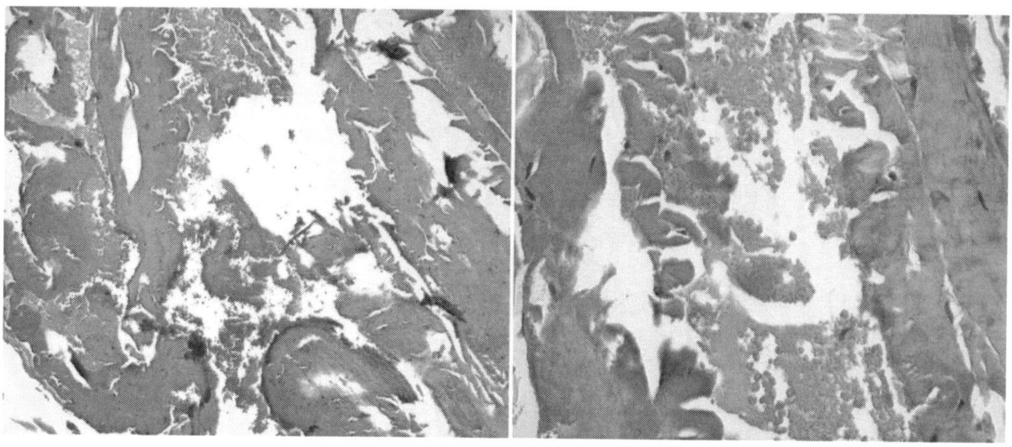

Figure 2-27. Intraosseous hemangiomas: It involves the accumulation of thin-walled blood vessels.

Treatment

- Mostly discovered by accident. Therefore, no treatment is needed. Some may regress spontaneously.
- Spinal compression: Surgery is required. Pre-operative embolization or angiography may also be needed.
- Painful or recurrent lesions in the vertebrae undergo radiotherapy/embolization.
- Vertebroplasty: It can treat pain but may not be effective for a long time.

DD

- Angiosarcoma: no fat, more infiltrative.
- Paget: The bone is enlarged, the end plate is thickened, and the trabeculae are less orderly.
- Metastasis: No fat or thickened trabeculae inside the lesion.
- LCH Compression fractures are rare for hemangiomas but are common in LCH. LCH has no internal fat.

- Intraosseous lipoma: Central or ring-like calcification is characterized by the absence of hemangiomas.

Bone-Like Tumor Lesions

Stress Fracture

- Fatigue Fx: Repetitive stress on a normal bone.
- Insufficiency Fx: Normal stress to the weak bone with osteoporosis, Paget or FD
- Strees fx
  - Metatarsals
  - Tarsus
  - T BIA (Proximal T-poster poster)
  - Recent history of increased activity
- The lucent line may be seen and is often perpendicular to the cortex
- The above line can be seen well in CT
- It has no soft tissue mass
- Can have a severe periosteal reaction.
- Can involve several adjacent bones.

Myositis Ossificans

Backgrounds

- trauma
- Burns
- Paraplegia
- Surgery
- Thermal brain damage
- hemophilia
- Ankylosing spondylitis
- DISH

Clinical Signs

- Patients may not remember therma.
- They may be asymptomatic or painful.
- It is usually found in the large muscles of the limbs.
- Bisphosphonate can play a prophylactic role.

Imaging

- Calcification: Seen 3 to 8 weeks after onset.
- It is calcified from the environment to the center.

Primary Lesion

- T1: Has a similar muscle signal
- T2 There is a large increase in signal and swelling.

The Lesion Is Ripe

- Isointese focuses on fat in the center.
- Dark in the environment. In both MRI views.
- Early stages with Sarcoma may be mistaken.
- CT: Helps see a plane of soft tissue between bone and ossicular mass, even if the lesion around the bone is complex.

Types of Hyperparathyroidism and Its Bone Lesions

- Primary: Usually caused by the parathyroid adenoma.
- Secondary: May be seen in chronic renal failure.

Imaging

- Diffuse demineralization. When hyperpara is diagnosed early.
- Focal destructive appearance similar to GCT when the lesion is diagnosed late.
- It is found in long bones, ribs, pelvis, and facial bones.
- With the treatment of parathyroid adenoma, lytic lesions begin to sclerosis.
- Lytic, expansile with even periosteal and multicellular reactions in the diaphysis or other areas of the bone.

Diagnostic Measures

- Calcium, Phosphorus, Alkaline Phosphatase, and PTH The presence of lytic lesions associated with hypercalcemia should lead the mind to hyperparathyroidism.

Microscopic Pathology

- It is generally similar to GCT with the following differences:
  - The evidence for bone metaplasia in the stroma is clearer.
  - Giant cells are slightly smaller than their GCT counterparts, and often accumulate nodular around foci of bleeding.
  - Stromal cells are thinner and more spindle-shaped.
  - Around the main lesion there is a clear osteoclastic and osteoblastic activity with peritrabecular fibrosis

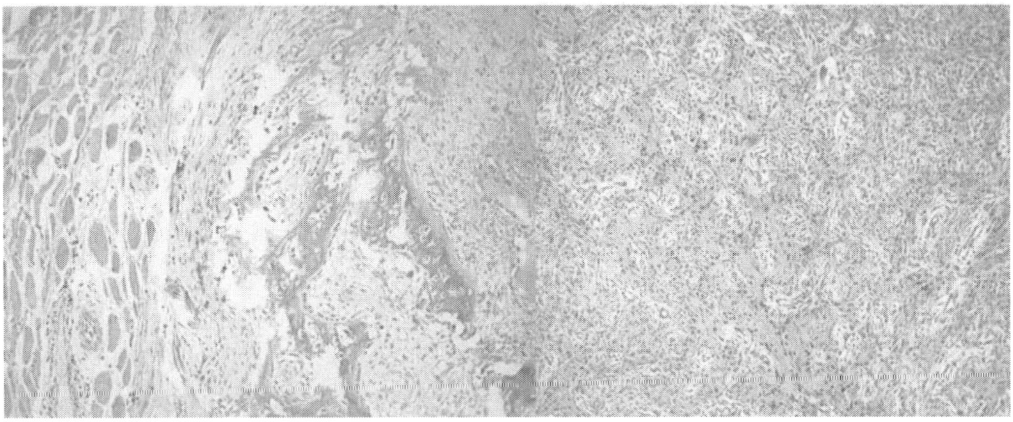

Figure 2-28. Myositis ossificans: The evidence for bone metaplasia in the stroma is clearer.

Giant cells are slightly smaller than their GCT counterparts, and often accumulate nodular around foci of bleeding .Stromal cells are thinner and more spindle-shaped.

MELORHEOSTOSIS

Definition

- Diffuse but localized thickening of the cortical bone.
- A benign dysplasia.

Common Place

- It is seen as mono-ostotic, or mono-malic.
- Rarely seen as monetary property.
- Most hyperostosis is seen in the long bone shaft.

Clinical Signs

- May be associated with venous arterial aneurysm, scleroderma, soft tissue hemangioma, neurofibroma, or osteo-poikilosis.
- 50% of patients do not show any signs of the disease until the age of 20.
- When symptomatic: Pain, limb deformity and contraction associated with muscle and tendon shortening, skin problems, and poor limb circulation can be seen.

Imaging

- It has the appearance of a wax dripping candle
- Confused with superficial osteosarcoma or osteochondroma.
- In the monomeric type, it has a sclerotomal distribution.
- Mineralized soft tissue masses are seen in 27% of patients near bone lesions or near joints.
- BS usually has an increase in absorption and in this case is differentiated from the bone island.

Osteonecrosis

Etiology

- trauma
- Corner disease
- Steroids
- Radiotherapy
- Hemoglobinopathies
- Chemotherapy
- Alcoholism
- Caison's disease
- Pancreatitis

Imaging

- Intramedullary bone infract is seen in metaphysis and diaphysis.
- AVN or bone infract epiphysis can lead to the collapse of the joint surface.
- X-ray: central lucency and sclerotic margin of serpentine Enchondromas, popcorn calcification in the center and peripheral lucency.

MRI

- BM edema in the early stages
- Double line T2
    - Internal high
    - Low environment

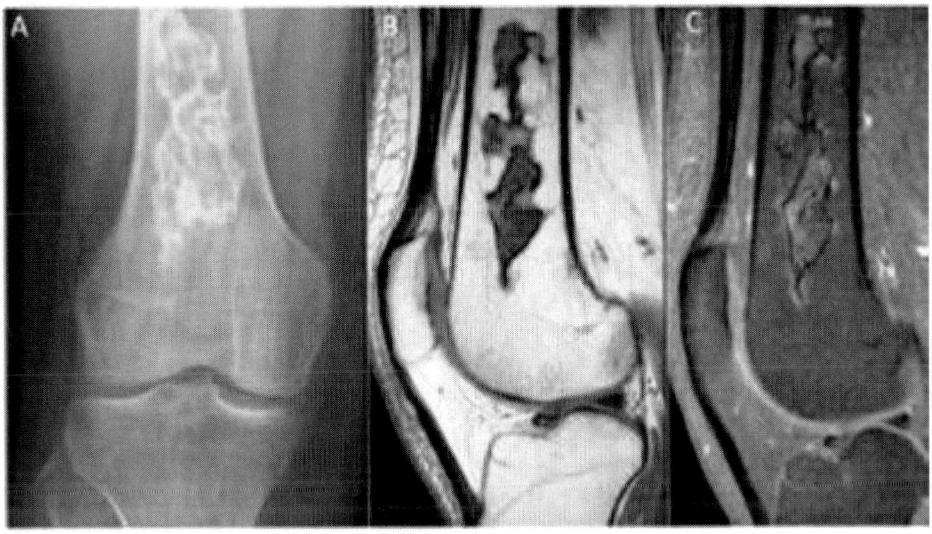

Figure 2-29. Osteonecrosis of distal femur.

Paget Disease

Another name: Osteitis deformans.

Epidemiology

- Under 50 is rare.
- Seen in 10% of the population over 80 years.
- Common in the UK and Australia.
- Rare in Chinese people.
- Men are equal to women or slightly more involved.

Etiology and Pathogenesis

- Leads to dilation and deformity.
- Bone remodeling is abnormal.
- Associated with viral paramyxovirus infection.

Common Place

- The pelvis is the most commonly involved area and is often involved unilaterally.
- Clinical signs.
- The finding may be accidental on the radiograph.
- Only 1% of patients develop extensive involvement and specific deformities.
- Typical Paget deformity is a large head, an outward curvature of the femur and tibia, and a dorsal hump.
- May be associated with bone pain, fractures, arthritis, deafness, increased head size, kidney stones, loose teeth, and high-efficiency heart failure.

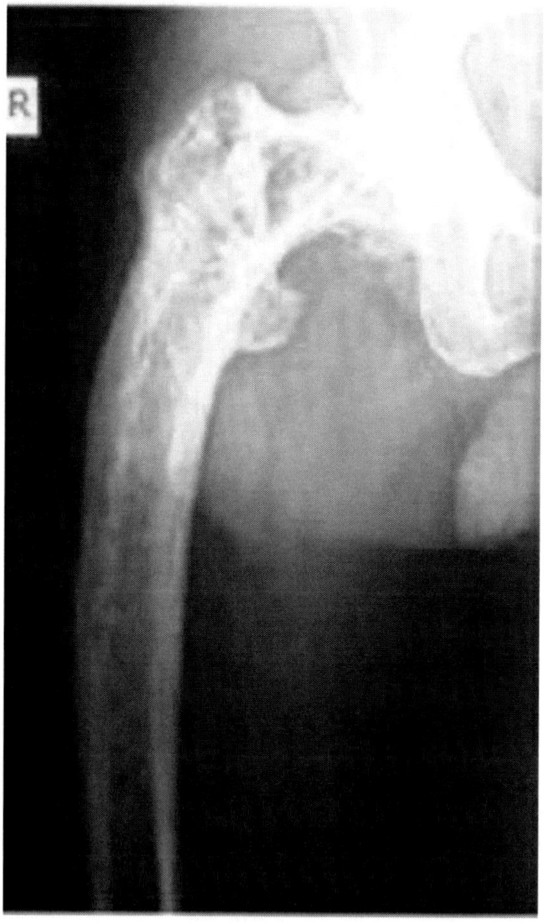

Figure 2-30. Paget disease causing coxa-vara deformity in right proximal femur.

Imaging

- The general radiological appearance is cotton wool with intermediate lucent areas.
- Acute phase: Bone resorption begins at the end of the long bones. The progressive margin of absorption is towards the diaphysis: as. Blade of gross or Flame.

- Exception in TIA: The lucent region is in the center of the diaphysis, without involving the end of the bone.
- The dormancy phase is characterized by bone deposition, thickening of the trabeculae and bone cortex, and overall bone enlargement.
- Osteoporosis circumscripta: The primary lesions of the skull are seen as lytic lesions, a circle with a definite margin.
- In areas with bone pairs, only one of the bones is involved.
- Bone scans usually increase absorption.

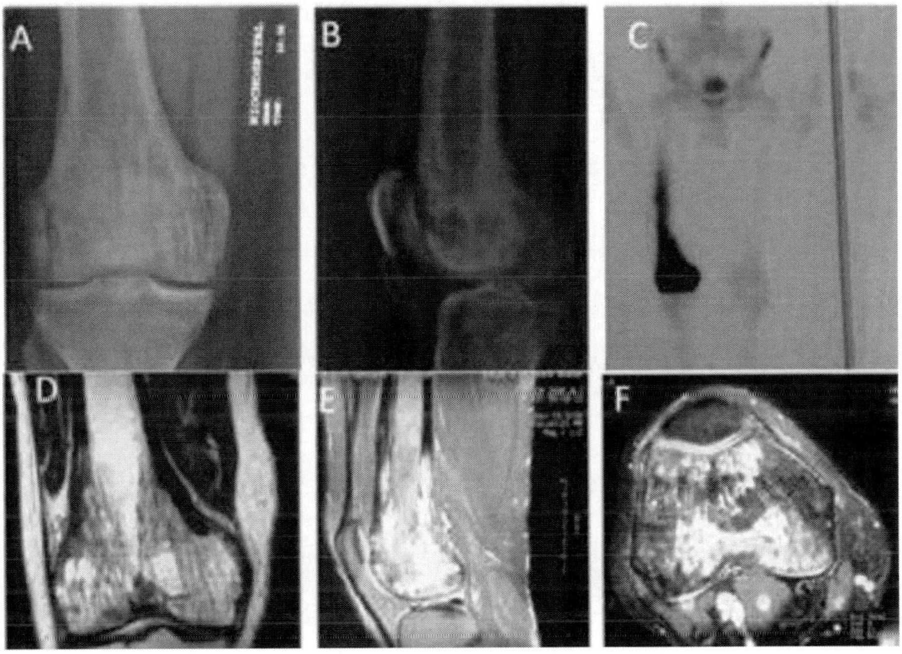

Figure 2-31. A and B: Thickened trabeculae C: an increase in uptake in bone scan D MRI T1 E and F MRI T2.

Microscopic Pathology

- Increased osteoclast activity with fibrosis and filling of intravascular spaces.
- Trabeculae are indigestible and have irregular mineralization with a mosaic appearance.
- Sclerosis is more common in the final phase.
- Different phases of the disease can be seen in different parts of a bone.

Treatment

- Medical treatment: Non-steroidal anti-inflammatory drugs, calcitonin, and bisphosphonates.
- Surgical treatment: treatment of deformities and pathological fractures.
- Bleeding during surgery can be very severe during surgery.
- Serum alkaline phosphatase and urinary pyridinium crosslink can be used to monitor disease activity.

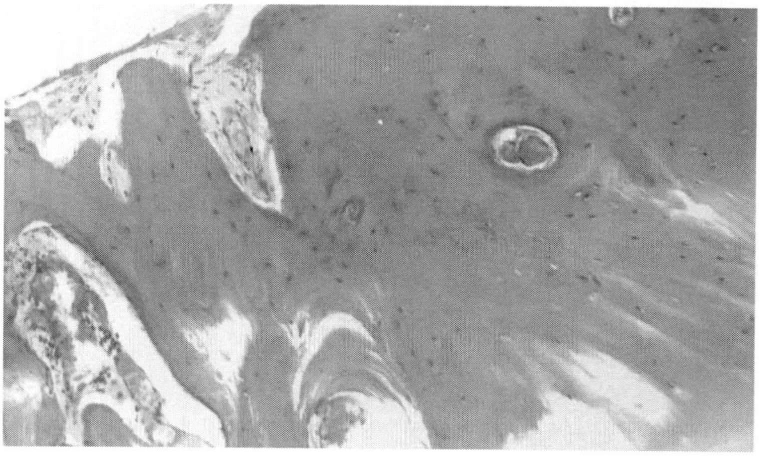

Figure 2-32. Paget disease: Irregularly thickened bony trabecula, Bone marrow is replaced by fibrovascular connective tissue.

Becoming Malignant

- Between 1 and 10%, depending on the extent of the conflict, becomes malignant.
- The most common sarcoma is osteosarcoma.
- It accounts for 20% of bone sarcomas over the age of 40.
- Its incidence increases with age.
- Pelvis, humerus, and femur are the most common areas of sarcoma.
- The lytic view is the dominant view of radiology.
- 5-year survival is 8% versus 50 to 65% in primary osteosarcoma.

PUBLIC OSTEOLYSIS

Definition

- Rapidly progressive osteolysis around the pubis.

Epidemiology

- It usually affects middle-aged or older women.

Radiography

- Bone slip in the pubis area.
- Bone fracture or fragmentation occurs later.
- Inflammation of the soft tissue around the bone slip area.
- It eventually occurs within the lysis area and in the soft tissue adjacent to sclerosis.

Microscopic Pathology

- There is ineffective and excessive bone call.
- Metaplastic cartilage is always seen and histological appearance may be predominant.
- Bone metaplasia is also commonly seen as immature woven bone formation.

Other

- It is important to make a mistake with chondrosarcoma.
- Underlying factors:
  - Trauma
  - Severe osteopenia

OSTEOLYSIS AFTER TRAUMA

Common Place

- Older women's pubis with osteopenia. Previously described.
- Distal clavicle of athletes, especially weightlifters.

Imaging

- It can look like a malignant tumor.

TUMORAL CALCINOSIS

Description

- Calcium deposition inside soft tissue in the form of a tumor without disturbance of calcium metabolism.

Epidemiology

- It is rare. It is seen in children, adolescents, and young adults. PK age is in the 2nd and 3rd decades.
- It is more common in girls than in boys.
- It is more common in blacks.
- May have two or more siblings in the family.

Location

- It is often multiple.
- It is usually found in the soft tissue around the joints, especially around the large joints: hip, shoulder, behind the elbow.
- Occasionally affects the knee and spine.
- It is very rare in the hands and feet.
- Bilateral and symmetrical involvement is common.
- It may occur in several generations of the family, as well as in siblings.
- Dominant autosomal inheritance has been suggested for the disease.

Clinical Signs

- Seen as an asymptomatic mass.
- May cause tenderness or pain.
- Hypercalcemia may be moderate to mild in many patients.
- Calcitriol levels may also be high.
- Key acid and alkaline phosphatase are normal.

Imaging

- A margin with a definite margin in the soft tissue adjacent to the large joints to the conglomerate pattern.
- Fluid levels are sometimes seen on radiographs, especially in larger and more chronic lesions.
- The foci of calcification are varying in size from a few millimeters to 1 to 2 centimeters.

Macroscopic Pathology

- A hard capsule mass that contains several nodules attached to each other.
- Cystic changes are commonly seen in some nodules.
- The nodules are filled with yellowish-gray or milky liquid.

Pathology Microscopic

- Large amorphous or granular calcium mass, sometimes centered with intermediate areas of calcified blades.

Differential Diagnosis

- Metabolic disorders with calcium deficiency (such as chronic renal failure or secondary hyperparathyroidism): Metabolic patients are typically older, have a history of underlying disorders, or show signs of generalized calcium deficiency.

- Other Calcium Level Disorders: In these diseases, calcium levels are typically abnormal. These conditions include primary hyperparathyroidism, hypervitaminosis D, alkaline milk syndrome, and scleroderma.

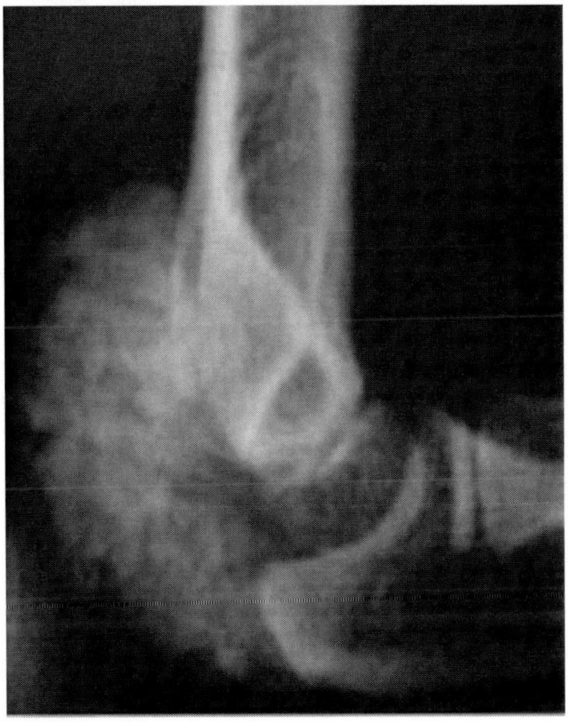

Figure 2-33. Tumoral calcinosis in elbow.

Treatment

- The treatment of choice is surgical removal of the lesion.
- Incomplete lesions recur.
- Chronic lesions can cause infection and abscesses.
- It is recommended that waste be removed as soon as possible when it is smaller and can be completely removed.
- Phosphorus-binding antacids and calcium deprivation: Recommended for lesions that are not technically removable.
- Radiotherapy, cortisone, low phosphate foods, aluminum hydroxide gels are ineffective in the treatment process.

TOPHACEOUS PSEUDOGOUT

Definition

- Calcium pyrophosphate dehydrate tumor crystal deposition disease. The term includes pseudo-gout, chondrocalcinosis and pyrophosphate arthropathy.

History

- McCarty was first described in 1962 in patients with symptoms similar to gout but without sodium urate crystals, and the disease was called pseudo-gout.
- Other names: Chondrocycosis and orthopathy Calcium pyrophosphate deposition.

Imaging

- It is a more or less calcified mass.
- The pattern of the calcification is granular or fluffy.
- Unlike ocular myositis, it does not have peripheral calcification.
- Pressure erosion is seen on adjacent bone.

Clinical Signs

- Average age: 60 years (30 to 86 years).

Common Place

- In the limbs.

Macroscopic Pathology

- It is a grayish-white mass with a more or less gypsum appearance.
- The average size of the lesion is 2 to 4 cm.

Pathology Microscopic

- It is cellular or low-cellular tissue containing small or large basophilic islets of calcium-containing substances.
- The crystals are rhomboid and short.
- They may rarely look like needle.
- Weak positive birefringence under polarized light microscope.
- Around the calcified areas, a large number of histiocytes and multinucleated Janet cells are seen, which is in the full cell part of the lesion.
- In the small cell section, the metaplastic chondroid tissue is seen.
- Chondroid cells can mimic malignant cartilage tumors.

Differential Diagnosis

- Chondrosarcoma: Macroscopically, pseudo-gout is a calcified gypsum mass that differs from the calcification in chondrosarcoma. The birefringent in a polarized microscope also helps differentiate most importantly.
- Synovial chondromatosis and synovial chondroma: No rhomboid crystals are seen inside the soft tissue of the indus.

Treatment

- May recur after incomplete or even complete removal.

Other

- Cleft multifocal calcification is clearly seen in the articular cartilage and intervertebral disc.

Tophaceous Gout

Epidemiology

- 90% is seen in men.
- PK is over 50 years old.
- If seen in women, it is typically after menopause.

Clinical Signs

- Many patients with hyperuricemia are asymptomatic, about 80%.
- 20% of patients with hyperuricemia have kidney stones or gouty arthritis attacks.
- In acute attacks of gout, monoarthritis or oligoarticular arthritis is seen.
- The joints of the foot or ankle are usually affected. The knee is also commonly involved. The small joints of the hand are then involved.
- Over time, painful attacks become longer and more frequent.
- In 50% of patients with gouty arthritis, there is a deposition of monosodium urate crystals called Tophi.
- The higher the uric acid level, the greater the tendency to form tophi.

Imaging

- Tophi formation occurs 3 to 40 years after a gout attack
- Gout on radiography is seen as a mass of non-calcified soft tissue around the joint with relatively common erosions of the surrounding bones.
- 20 to 30% of Tophi are calcified

Macroscopic Pathology

- It is a white to yellow gypsum nodular area surrounded by interstitial fibrous tissue.
- Smaller lesions: show urate crystalline deposits.
- Larger and more chronic lesions: show a multilobular structure with fibrosis and calcification.

Microscopic Pathology

- Acupuncture crystals with strong negative birefringence under a polarized microscope are characteristic of monosodium urate crystals.
- These crystals float freely or are present inside leukocyte cells.

- Inside the tophi, monosodium urate crystals are seen as multicenter radial sediments surrounded by amorphous matter mats, lipids, and protein debris.
- The pattern of crystal deposition is multilobular or nodular and may be calcified.
- Stromal tissue includes interstitial histocytes and multinucleated giant cells.

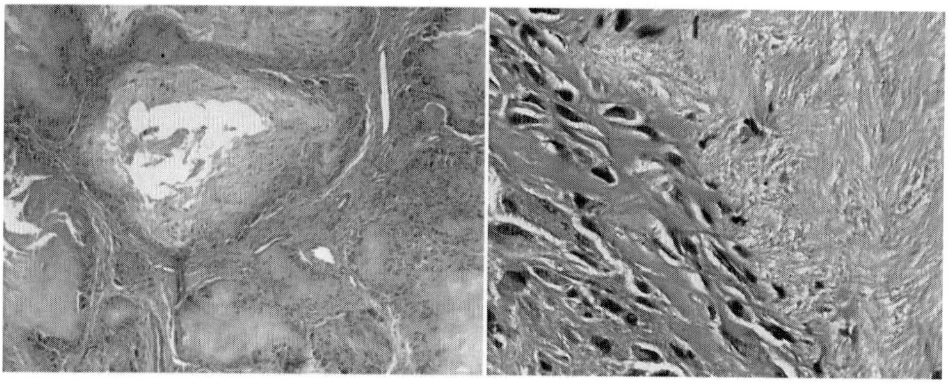

Figure 2-34. Tophaceous Gout: Amorphous material with granulomatous reaction.

CHRONIC RECURRENT MULTIFOCAL OSTEOMYELITIS CRMO

Definition

- It is a rare type of osteomyelitis that affects children and young adults.

Epidemiology

- It is more common in children and young adults.

Common Place

- It is common in metaphyses of long bones and clavicle.
- It is found in tibia, femur, clavicle, and fibula, respectively.
- Sometimes seen symmetrically.

Clinical Signs

- Pain, local swelling, and fever develop gradually.

Imaging

- They are seen as multiple metaphysical centers outside the center. Lytic lesions are associated with sclerosis.

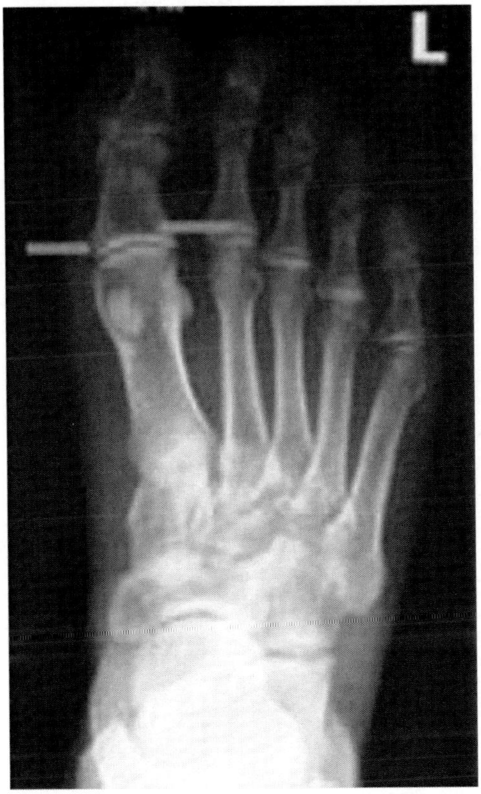

Figure 2-35. Erosions around the joint in gout.

Bone Scan

- Helps to find other focal points involved.

MRI

- There is no soft tissue involvement. Thus it is differentiable from malignancy.

Lab Tests

- ESR is often high.
- ASO can be high. Some have linked the previous throat infection and increased ASO to CRMO

Microscopic Pathology

- Primary lesions: Neutrophilic infiltration in the bone marrow. Accumulation of neutrophils can show the appearance of an abscess.
- Bone uptake and the presence of large numbers of osteoclasts are also common.

- Long-term lesions: have fibrosis and obvious lymphocytic infiltration.
- The presence of new reactive bone is obvious at this stage.
- Neutrophil-containing granulomas with a rim of epithelioid histocytes without bone necrosis may also be present.
- The results of bacterial, viral, and fungal cultures as well as specific staining for infectious organisms are always negative.

Differential Diagnosis

- Osteosarcoma: Involves metaphysis and is common in young adults and children (similar to CRMO).
- Ewings sarcomas: Especially when CRMOs affect the clavicle are similar. A biopsy helps to distinguish CRMO from osteosarcoma and Ewings sarcoma.
- Bone lymphoma: The late stage of CRMO, which is accompanied by marked infiltration of lymphocytes, can be confused with lymphoma. Bone lymphoma is almost never seen in young people. Also, CRMO should be multi-focal by definition. Also, a permeative lesion containing lymphocytes in a patient older than 40 years is highly unlikely to be chronic osteomyelitis.

Treatment and Course of the Disease

- Symptomatic treatment is with nonsteroidal anti-inflammatory drugs and pamidronate.
- Pamidronate can cause spinal remodeling.
- In general, the outcome of the disease is good.
- Some patients may have a stable illness for a long time.
- In a minority of patients, the disease may be prolonged and severe.

Other

- Associated with palmar-plantar pustulosis.

Bone Amyloidosis Description

Local amyloid deposition in bone.

Epidemiology

It is seen in the elderly. The age of onset is similar to the age of onset of myeloma types of:

- Primary: Very rare.
- Secondary: The most common type of amyloidosis that affects the skeleton is secondary to multiple myeloma. Then there is secondary amyloidosis to renal failure.

Clinical Signs

- Amyloid deposition in bone exposes a person to pathological fractures, especially in weight-bearing bones.
- It can cause symptoms by putting pressure on organs such as the spinal cord.
- It mostly covers the skull and spine.
- Pathology M. Chiroscopy.

- Amorphous eosinophilic deposition is seen within stromal tissue and around blood vessels.
- Amyloid deposits are typically metachromatic and have a positive staining with congo red and crystal violet.
- Congo red staining under polarized light is the most sensitive type of staining, in which case they take on green birefringence.
- Giant cells and mononuclear histocytes and plasma cells are also present.

Subchondral Cyst

- Very common
- Seen in DJD
- With the entry of synovium and joint fluid due to increased intra-articular pressure through cartilaginous defects into the subchondral bone is created
- Typically small in size and have a sclerotic margin.
- They can also extend into the bone shaft.
- They are more common in the elderly
- MRI
  - In T1 it has a low or dark signal.
  - In T2 it has a high or clear signal

DD

- Chondroblastoma
- Metastasylytic
- GCT
- Chondrosarcoma clear cell
- Langerhans cell histiocytosis
- The presence of DJD in the joint differentiates these lesions from the subchondral cyst

Chapter 3

Benign Aggressive Bone Lesions

Giant Cell Tumor (GCT)

Definition

Local aggressive neoplasms which have single-nucleated elliptical cells along with multinucleated giant cells.

Epidemiology

- It accounts for 4 to 5% of all primary bone tumors.
- The most common age is 20 to 55 years of age.
- 70% is observed in 20-40 years of age.
- Mostly common in the third decade.
- It is generally a little more common in women.
- Benign type: 1.5 times more common in women than men.
- Aggressive type: 3 times more common in men than women.

Types

- Primitive
- Secondary to another tumor

Site

- Mostly found in long bones (75 to 90%) and more around the knee.
- It is, respectively, more common in the distal femur, proximal tibia, and distal radius.
- The most common area of the axial skeleton involvement is the sacrum.
- It starts from the metaphysis and then expands to the epiphysis.

- Outside the sacrum in the spine, it engages the body of the vertebrae.
- In 1 to 2% of the case, it may be multifocal at the same time or at separate intervals.

Signs

- Most of the patients have progressive pain, initially during exercise and then they have pain event in the rest time.
- Pain is rarely severe unless there is a pathological fracture.
- Swelling, tenderness, decreased range of motion may exist too.
- There is a pathological fracture in 10 to 30% of the initial examinations. Some reports state this to be from 5 to 10%.

Imaging

- As a lucent, eccentric lesion, the epiphysis is tangent to the subchondral bone.
- The cortex usually raises or gets perforated. Cortex perforation is observed in 20 to 50% of the cases.
- The periosteal reaction is observed in the area of the fracture and only scarcely.
- Tumors can be observed in the metaphyses of the patients with open physis.
- Zone of transition may be indistinctive.
- The tumor side facing the diaphysis is closer to the midline than the tumor side facing the epiphysis.

CT

Seeing the thinned cortex, new periosteal ossification, fluid-fluid surfaces, and proving the absence of matrix calcification are useful. Soft tissue masses are observed on CT scans in 44% of the cases.

MRI

- The best modality is to see the tumor spread into the joint with soft tissue.
- Low signal in T_1 and high signal in T_2.
- In 20% of the cases, the fluid-fluid level is observed on MRI due to secondary ABC.
- The signal may be moderate at T_2. The reason for the low or moderate signal in T_2 is fibrosis and intra-tumor hemosiderin.
- Sometimes the signal increase in T2 can be observed due to cystic tumors or due to the formation of secondary ABC.
- In tumors with too much prostaglandin around the lesion, a decrease in bone marrow signal, and in contrast an increased uptake can be observed due to an inflammatory response.
- The recurrence of the lesion is nodular rather than diffuse.

BS

- Most often have an increase in absorption a delay in the blood pool phase.
  Dount sign: refers to the increased absorption of tumor margins due to hyperemia or reactive osteogenesis.
- Sometimes there is an increase in absorption in the adjacent joint due to congestion and should not be mistaken with the spread of the tumor into the joint.

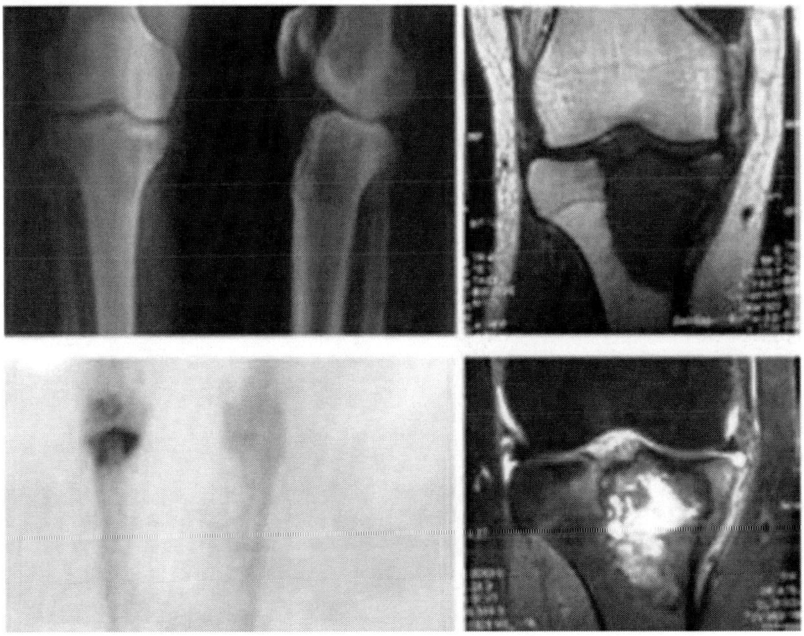

Figure 3-1. Giant cell tumor (GCT) of the medial tibia plateau. Top left: plain radiograph of anterior-posterior. A radiolucent lesion with a marked margin in the proximal tibial epiphysis. Top right: T1 MRI: The lesion is observed with a decrease in signal. Bottom left: Bone scan. No increase in uptake is observed in the tumor area. Bottom right. MRI view of T2 fat suppressor. The lesion is moderate to high.

Malignancy Potential

Benign metastasizing: 2 to 5% of benign GCTs have lung metastasis. Indeed, it is a kind of implantation rather than real metastasis, as the histology of metastasis is not malignant. It is observed 3-4 years after the initial diagnosis. Most radiologically lesions include soft tissue lesions, distal radius lesions, or lesions with more than one recurrence.

- Malignant transformation does not need manipulation at first, sometimes it can become malignant on its own, though it is very.
- Secondary malignant transformation: this is observed at the site of a previously treated tumor, usually with radiotherapy. With radiotherapy over Gy40 can be observed in 29% of the cases. This is observed within 5-8 years after radiotherapy. The prognosis is worse.

Giant cell sarcoma: Sarcomas contain giant cells. The prognosis is bad. They are not giant cell tumors.

Macroscopic Pathology

- It is observed in form of a soft reddish-brown flesh mass with yellow areas.
- Brown areas are caused by macrophages containing hemosiderin.
- Bleeding, necrosis, and cyst formation are common in the tumor. The first two are more common in weight-bearing bones.
- Growth usually continues until it reaches the articular cartilage.
- Bone dilation and thinning of the bone cortex are more common than being intact.
- The most common area for pathological fractures is the subchondral bone.

Microscopic Pathology

- Tumor stroma is moderately vascular.
- There are single-nucleated spindle cells along with multi-nucleated giant cells, sometimes with 50 to 100 nuclei.
- The nuclei of giant cells and spindle cells are similar. This feature helps to differentiate this tumor from other tumors with giant cells.
- Areas of spindle cells, reactive ossification and foamy macrophages might exist in the tumor.
- After simple curettage, it is more than 50%.
- Recurrence is observed typically in the first three years.

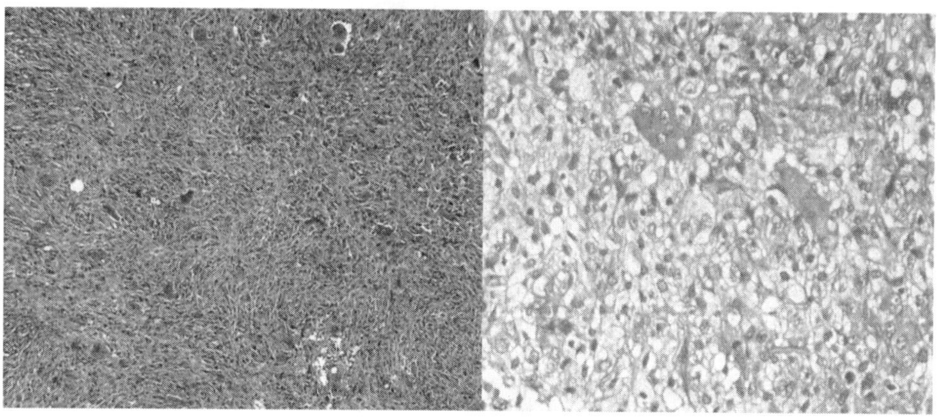

Figure 3-2. Giant cell tumor: The nuclei of giant cells and spindle cells are similar. This feature helps to differentiate this tumor from other tumors with giant cells.

Treatment

- In the new studies, after extensive curettage, recurrence is 5 to 15%.
- Extensive curettage and bone grafts are the preferred treatment.
- Some prefer cementing.
- The advantages of cement over bone grafting is reducing the recurrence because of heat generated and toxicity of cement monomers, faster patient initiation, and easier diagnosis of recurrence.
- The radiolucent line is not considered thinner than two millimeters around the incense cement.
- Recurrence is diagnosed as dilated lytic areas in the bone.

- Recurrence within the soft tissue is as swelling or calcification.
- Long follow-up is recommended given the recurrence/metastasis .every three months up to two years , then every six months in the third year, and then annually after the third year. Clinical examination of the tumor site and tumor site radiograph and chest radiograph are necessary measures in any follow-up.
- Ct scan is suggested if there are any abnormal changes observed on the chest radiograph.
- In some cases, stage 3 resection and reconstruction might be required from the start and curettage may be ineffective.
- These cases are treated by resection and hemicondylar allograft or hinge prosthesis in tumors around the knee and autograft using proximal fibula (arthroplasty or arthrodesis) in the distal radius.
- In insignificant bones (distal ulna and proximal fibula), resection is used without reconstruction.
- Radiotherapy or embolization or both are used for non-operable tumors in the spine or pelvis.
- Resection has to be used for lung metastases.
- Recurrence treatment is like treating a primary tumor. After the biopsy, the tumor is still benign, curettage, or resection or resection alone is performed.
- Radiotherapy is associated with the risk of sarcoma.

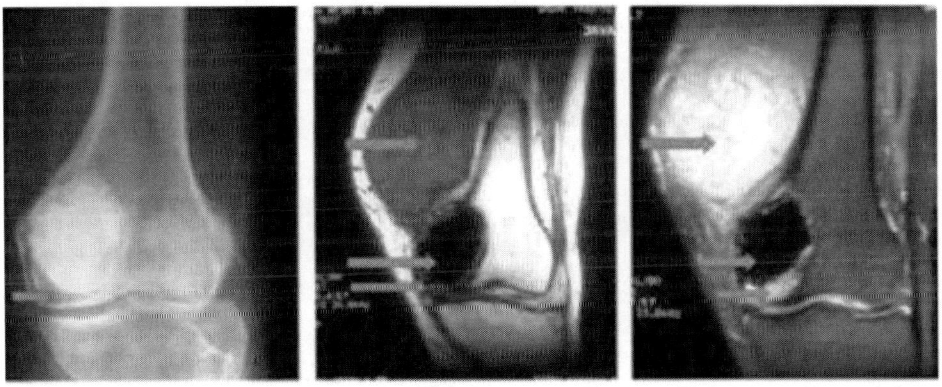

Figure 3-3. Timor giant cell recurrence. In plain radiography (left figure), the arrow shows a recurrence under the bone cement. In MRI T_1 (middle figure), and T_2 (right figure), arrows from top to bottom show recurrence within the soft tissue, bone cement, and recurrence below the bone cement.

Other

- Some multifocal cases are associated with Paget.
- Histological grade does not matter in terms of prognosis.

DD

ABC

After puberty, it can reach the subarticular end of the bone. At lower age, we do not have a solid component in ABC (Except in rare cases of solid ABC)

Brown Tumor

They have other symptoms of hyper-parathyroid disease.

- Subchondral cyst: has a sclerotic margin. The signal increase in T_2 is due to the internal fluid. Accompanying DJD is observed in the joint.
- Metastasis, myeloma is common in older ages.
- Brodie abscess: it has an extensive sclerosis border. In T_2, a large signal increase is observed due to surrounding edema.
- Clear sell chondrosarcoma: It is rounder, has chondroid calcification and is epiphyseal.

GIANT CELL REPARATIVE GRANULOMA

Definition

- The heterogeneous group of benign lesions including reactive and turmoral lesions.they are characterized by multinucleated giant cell masses in fibrous stroma containing reactive ossification.

Epidemiology

- Peak age is in the second decade of life. The most common age is 10-25 years old.

Site

- Craniofacial bones have the highest prevalence like Mandela and Maggila.
- Small bones of the hands and feet are the second most common.
  - They are common in metaphysis and diaphysis.
  - The lesion is observed centrally with severe bone dilation and thinning of the cortex without destruction.
  - Epiphyseal involvement can be observed after puberty, always due to the spread of metaphyseal involvement.

CHONDROBLASTOMA

Definition

An invasive benign tumor encompasses the proliferation of immature cartilage cells along with foci of cartilage matrix that typically involve the long bones of the immature bone of immature individuals.

Epidemiology

- The most common age is 15-25 years in the second decade.
- 10% happens in the fifth and subsequent decades.
- 50% happens before skeletal puberty.
- It is rare. It accounts for less than 1% of bone tumors.

Site

- The epiphysis is involved.
- 75% is found in long bones.
- The commonest areas involved are the distal femur, proximal tibia, proximal humerus, and proximal femur.
- The two extremities (pelvis, calcaneus, talus, patella, and scapula) are mostly involved.
- A rare lesion that can affect the patella.
- Multifocal lesions have been reported as well.
- It is rarely reported within metaphysis. This is usually more aggressive.
- It is observed in atypic area in older patients.

Clinical Signs

- Pain is the initial symptom.
- Joint dryness (because of inflammatory changes) may exist.
- Joint effusion is observed in 30% of the cases.
- Deafness, dizziness, and tinnitus due to temporal bone tumors may exist.

Imaging

- It is observed as a lucent, a round or oval lesion with a distinct margin with a size of 3-6 cm in the epiphysis or apophysis.
- It tends to be central in the epiphysis as opposed to GCT that is extra central.
- The margin of sclerosis is observed in 60% of the cases.
- There is a narrow Zone Of Transition (ZOT) in 60% of the cases.
- The chondroid matrix is present in 1/3 cases as a ring or arc calcification within the lesion.
- The physis is open in 70% of the cases.
- It is typically non-expansile. If there is expansion, chondroblastoma with ABC has to be considered.
- Fluid-Fluid level on Ct / MRI has to be associated with ABC.
- 15 to 20% associated with secondary ABC.

MRI

- Low T_1.
- It is heterogeneous high T_2. Because of the cellular matrix inside the tumor, its heterogeneously increases the signal (unlike the uniformly clear signal at 2_T observed in chondroma).
- MRI shows a wider area of the actual size of the tumor because of bone marrow edema.

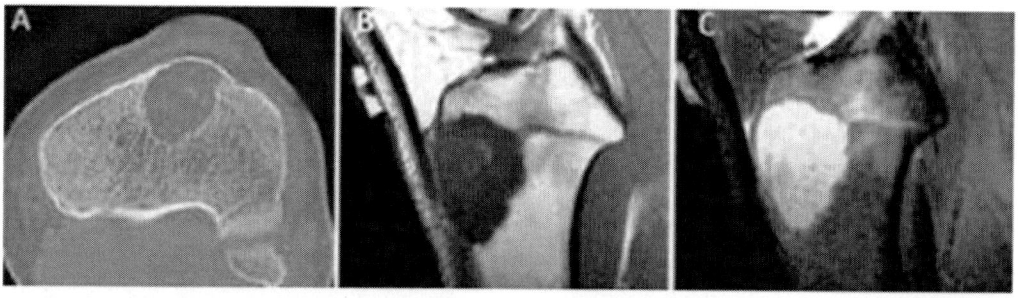

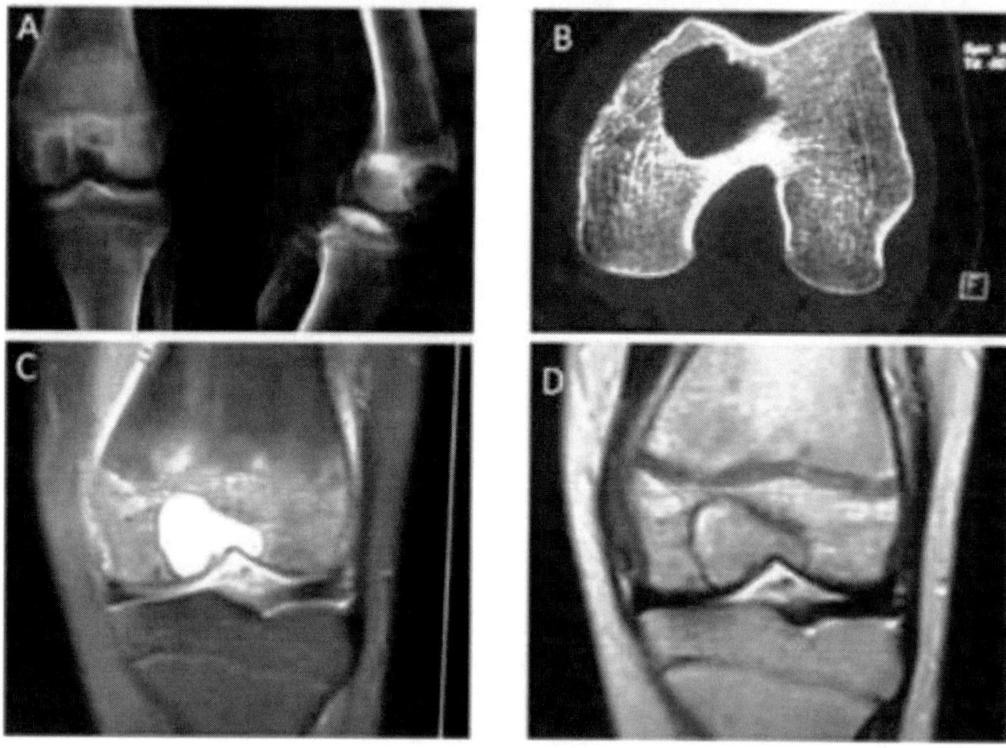

Figure 3-4. Radiography of anterior-posterior of the knee, a small lesion with marked margins in the distal femoral epiphysis. B CT scan of the axial. C. T2 coronary MRI shows a lesion with increased signal in the epiphysis and second bone surrounding. D MRI T1 coronary view of the lesion is observed with a reduced signal.

Aggressive type: can pass through the growth plate and enter the joint or metaphysis. It has a soft texture and a thick periosteal reaction.

It rarely becomes chondrosarcoma.

- Pulmonary metastasis without malignant cells may be associated with previous surgical treatment (due to cell implantation).

Macroscopic Pathology

- It has a brittle, yellow appearance with white calcified foci.
- It may have cystic changes or be completely cystic except for the thin solid margin around the tumor.

Microscopic Pathology

- Numerous chondroblasts are observed along with multinucleated giant cells.
- The cells and their nuclei are round or oval. The nucleus of the cells has a longitudinal gap.
- Calcification in the form of chicken wire can be observed around individual single-celled cells. In this case, a thin layer of calcification surrounds the cell like a small wire.

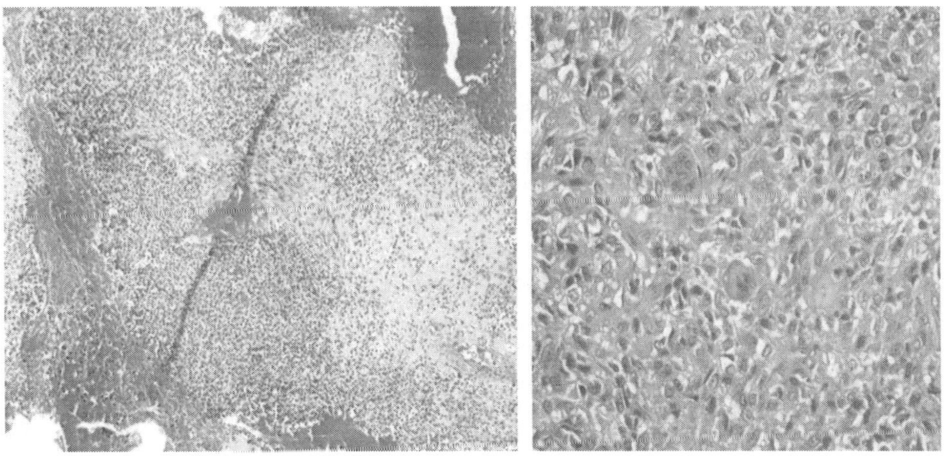

Figure 3-5. Chondroblastoma: Numerous chondroblasts are observed along with multinucleated giant cells. Cells and their nuclei are round or oval.

Treatment

- Curettage with bone graft is sufficient.
- The recurrence is 10 to 15% and is typically observed in the first 2 years.
- Recurrence is more common if the tumor is in the atypical region or is associated with ABC.
- Recurrent curettage treatment is accompanied by bone grafting.

Other

- Codman's tumor is another name for it.
- In old age (elderly) it is observed in atypical areas.
- Temporal bone involvement is observed in people over forty.
- It behaves more aggressively than long bone in flat bone.
- The metaphyseal type can be more aggressive.

- Tuberculosis, especially in developing countries, has to be included in the differential diagnosis of chondroblastoma.
- The main long-term problem in these patients is osteoarthritis of the adjacent joint, observed in up to 5% of the cases.

DD

- GCT: Located on the scar (remnant) phase: it goes into the epiphysis and metaphysis. It is more eccentric than chondroblastoma.
- Osteomyelitis: It does not have sclerosis rim.
- Clear Cell Chondrosarcoma: It is observed in older people, the tumor is larger in size and more likely to spread beyond the epiphysis.
- Subchondral cyst: It has DJD. It does not have a chondroid matrix.
- Eosinophilic grnuloma: It is observed as epiphyseal leukemia in children and young adults and differs in microscopy.

CHONDROMYXOID FIBROMA

Definition

- Benign cartilaginous tumor has immature myxoid tissue with primary cartilage differentiation.

Epidemiology

- It is the rarest cartilage tumor.
- The peak age is in the second and third decades.
- $M \div F = 1 \cdot 5 \div 1$

Site

- Proximal tibia is the most common site involved.
- Distal femur is the second most common.
- It can also be observed in the ribs, feet, and hands.
- The ilium is the most common flat bone involved.
- It is metaphyseal. It rarely passes physis.

Clinical Signs

- Symptoms include progressive slow pain, tenderness, swelling, and limited movement.
- The patient may have pain for years before being diagnosed.

- It is rarely asymptotic (pelvic ribs).
- Painless swelling in the hands or feet can be the patient's main complaint.

Imaging

- It is completely lytic. The thin sclerotic margin (thinner than NOF) is metaphyseal.
- Calcification is rare (7 to 13%), except in superficial lesions that can have a lot of calcification.
- It is Eccentric in the metaphysis. Its longitudinal axis is parallel to the longitudinal axis of the bone.
- It is usually accompanied by a cortical bubbling sign. Severe protrusion of the cortex is a sign of secondary ABC mounting on the chondromyxoid fibroma.
- On MRI it is dark at T_1 and bright at T_2.

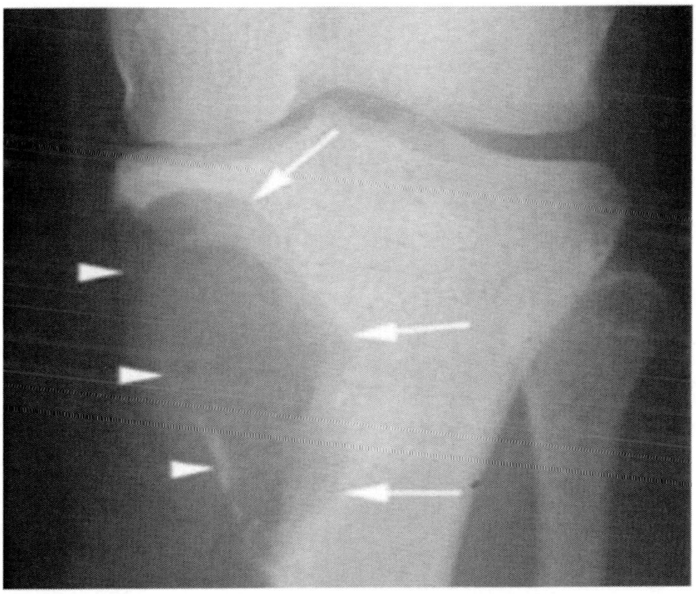

Figure 3-6. Chypromyxoid fibroma. The arrows show the tumor and the arrowheads the dilation of the cortex.

Malignancy Potential

- It is rare.

Macroscopic Pathology

- Stiff, white-gray lobulated mass with marked margins.
- It is always worn with a healthy periosteum even when the cortex is not observed on the radiograph.

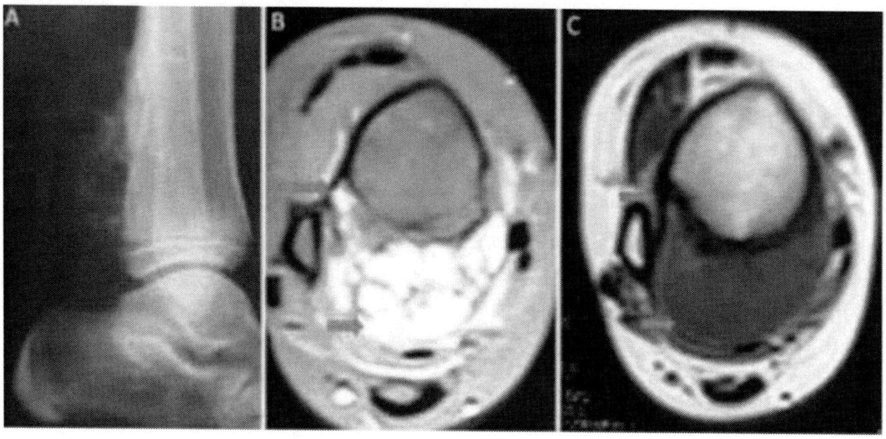

Figure 3-7. Chondromycoid fibroma of juxta cortical. The left side is observed on a plain radiograph of the lesion in the posterior tibial cortex. In MRI T2 (middle figure) and T1 (right figure). The upper arrows show the bone cortex and the lower ones the extra-bony component of the tumor.

Microscopic Pathology

- It is lobulated.
- It contains loose myxoid areas in the center of the lobulated and fibrotic areas with more cells in the peripheral areas.
- Chondroid tumor background, although specific areas of hyaline cartilage are rarely observed.
- Mitosis is very rare.
- Histologically, it is similar to chondroblastoma.

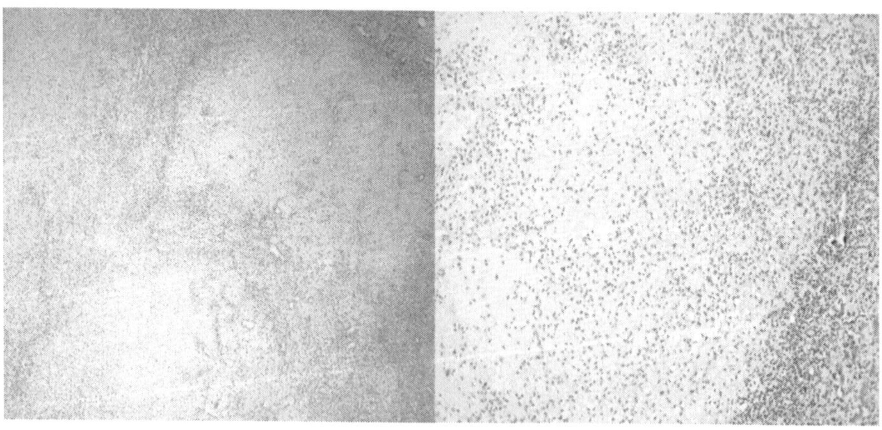

Figure 3-8. Chondromyxoid fibroma: It contains loose myxoid areas in the center of the lobulated and fibrotic areas with more cells in the peripheral areas.

Treatment

- Extensive curettage and bone graft or wide excision is the standard treatment.
- 15 to 25% local recurrence is observed with curettage: on average 20%.
- Recurrence treatment is reoperation.

DD

- Chondroblastoma: It is epiphyseal. Chondroblastoma is hard to differentiate in its pathology.
- NOF: It is more common, the sclerotic rim is thicker, it has no cortical bubbling.
- FD: Has a ground glass view. It is central.
- ABC: Liquid-liquid surfaces.
- GCT: Usually has no sclerotic rim and extends to the joint surface.
- Chondrosarcoma: More aggressive appearance, more likely cortical destruction, more soft tissue component, and more chondroid matrix.

Miscellaneous on the Comparison of Fibroid Chondromyxoid and Chondroblastoma

- CMF and chondroblastoma are usually stage 2 or stage 3 of the enneking classification. Chondroblastoma is usually more painful than CMF.
- Pain is the most common complaint in Chondrobblastoma then a decrease in ROM in the foot area, the subchondral fracture can be observed as common.
- In CMF, pain is more common than an accidental lesion. It is persistent pain. The next manifestation is inflammation.
- In chondroblastoma, the lesion is usually less than 4 cm in size and can pass the physis.
- Noticeably, chondroblastoma is epiphyseal and chondromyxoid fibroma is metaphyseal.
- For reading more:
- SAAOS/4No:/21vol/2013April

OSTEOBLASTOMA

Definition

- Osteoblastic tumor which is a rare disease closely related to osteoid osteoma.

Epidemiology

- It is rarer than osteoid osteoma.

The most common age is between 10 and 30 years.

- Males are 3 times more likely to be affected than females.
- Some references state that, like osteoarthritis, men are affected twice women.

Common Site

- 40 to 50% of the cases are in the spine (posterior element) and sacrum.
- The femur, jaw, and tibia are in the second most common site.
- It is mostly nodular, rarely cortical.

Signs

- Pain is the most common symptom. The pattern of pain may be similar to pain in an osteoid osteoma but the pain is less severe.
- Scoliosis, back spasm, and neurological symptoms can be observed in spinal cord injury.
- Symptoms of pressure on the spinal cord are more common in the thoracic spine and pressure on nerve roots in lumbar spine.
- Symptoms may exist 1 to 2 years before diagnosis because of the slow growth of the tumor.
- Toothache can be observed if it is in the jaw.
- Osteoid Osteoma does not respond well to aspirin.
- Osteomalacia can occur due to the release of chemicals that disrupt the proximal tubules of the kidney (tumor-induced osteomalacia).

Imaging

- Typically a bone lesion in the posterior element of a spine in a young person.
- It is similar to an osteoid osteoma, but the nidus is larger than two centimeters. Osteoid osteoma's nidus is less than 1.5 cm. A lytic lesion with a definite margin with sclerosis has a surrounding reaction.
- It can be completely lytic, sclerotic, or a mixture of both.
- It is similar to ABC in Spine. Lytic is expanding.
- Aggressive osteoblastoma is an aggressive lesion with a periosteal reaction.
- Juxtactacortical is very rare.
- It is usually 2 to 3 cm, sometimes in the giant type, it may be larger than 15 cm.
- 30% of the cases have internal calcification.
- Unlike osteoid osteoma, the component can have soft tissue. This condition is rare in other areas except in the spine.
- 66% occur in the cortex, 33% in the medullary bone.

CT

- The best imaging modality.
- Useful for spine, nidus and central calcification lesions.

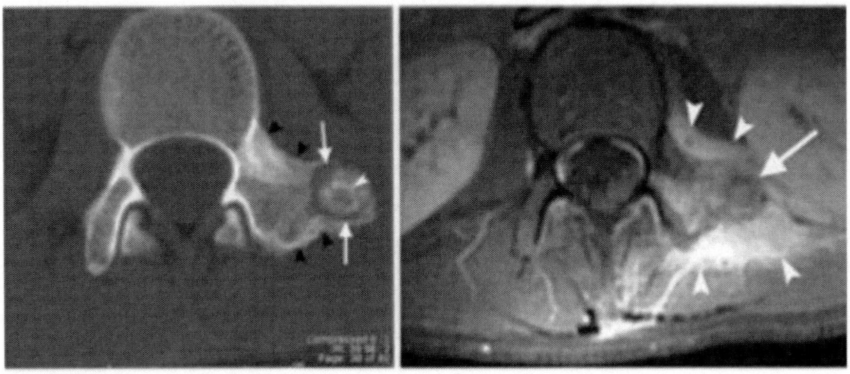

Figure 3-9. Osteoblastoma is the transverse appendage of the vertebra. Left: In a CT scan, the axial arrow shows Nidus, the black arrowhead shows cortical hypertrophy, and the white arrowhead show intracellular calcification. Right: Axial T2 MRI cut with contrast. The arrow shows Nidus and the arrowhead show the surrounding soft tissue which both of them show an increase in uptake.

MRI

- It is possible to have a Fluid-Fluid level view similar to ABC.
- It shows soft tissue involvement and BM.
- It is useful to show pressure on the spinal cord.

BS

- It has a sharp increase in absorption in all three phases.

Malignancy Potential

- Aggressive type has a more concerning appearance in histology.

Macroscopic Pathology

- The appearance of Nidus is like the nidus of osteoid osteoma.
- Nidus has fragile red granular tissue that may bleed profusely during curettage and can be easily removed from the surrounding bone.
- Bone margins may have severe dilation.
- Bleeding and secondary cystic changes may happen in the tumor that alter the macroscopic appearance of the tumor.

Microscopic Pathology

- Histology is similar to osteoid osteoma.
- It is an intertwined network of bony trabeculae evenly distributed within a loose fibrous stroma with abundant arteries.
- Osteoblastic monolayers are evident around the bony trabeculae.
- This feature helps to differentiate between osteoblastoma and osteosarcoma.
- Giant cells are observed as multinucleated.

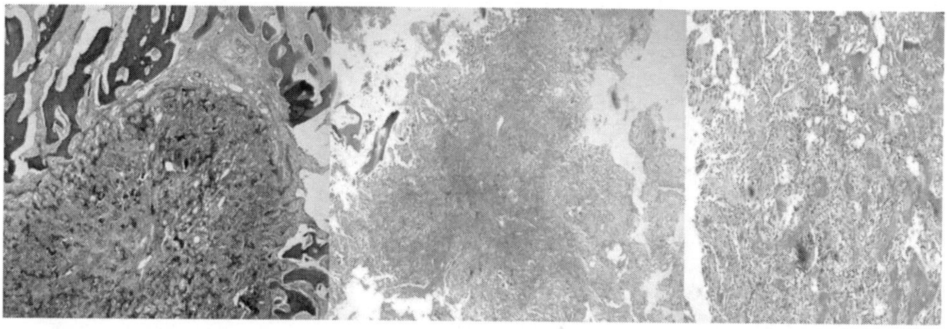

Figure 3-10. Osteoblastoma: It is an intertwined network of bony trabeculae evenly distributed within a loose fibrous stroma with abundant arteries. Giant cells are observed as multinucleated.

Treatment

- Extensive curettage or marginal excision and bone graft are the standard treatment.
- Some writers suggest adjuvant radiotherapy for spinal tumors due to the difficulties of reoperation in the site of recurrence.
- Others argue that incomplete-removed lesions sometimes remain asymptomatic.
- Most writers oppose radiotherapy and suggest it only in symptomatic, inoperable cases.
- It usually has a recurrence of 10 to 15%.
- 50% of recurrence is observed in the aggressive type.
- Unlike osteoid osteoma, osteoarthritis does not go away on its own, and osteoid osteoma pain is not solved with NSAIDs.
- Unlike osteoids, osteoma observation is not an option for treatment because the lesion is constantly growing.
- Transformation to sarcoma has been reported, which is more common in patients who went through radiotherapy.
- In the follow-up, the patient should have a tumor site and chest radiograph.

DD

- ABC: It has no internal mineralization. Secondarily, ABC can mount on Osteoblastoma in 10 to 40% of the cases.
- Osteoid osteoma: The nidus is less than two centimeters.
- Osteosarcoma: it includes soft-tissue component.
- Brody abscess: may have a sinus tract or adjacent abscess.

Malignant Aggressive Osteoblastoma

- It is the boundary between osteoblastoma and osteosarcoma
- Tends to local recurrence but does not metastasize.
- Osteoblastoma is aggressive in 25% of the cases. It has typical atrial cells, abundant mitosis, and multinucleated giant cells.
- It can be differentiated from normal osteoblastoma through pathology. The presence of epithelioid osteoblasts that cover the bony trabeculae is the main difference between the aggressive type and the normal type.

- It is usually observed as a lytic lesion with sclerotic margins. There is severe bone dilation.
- The major difference with normal osteoblastoma in radiography is the size of the lesion: larger than 4 cm in the aggressive type.

Langerhans Cell Histiocytosis (LCH)

Definition

Cell proliferation with Langerhans cells features with appearance of CD1a and CD207 in immunohistochemistry and Birbeck granules in electron microscopy.

Other Names

- Eosinophilic granoma, histiocytosis

Epidemiology

- It is relatively rare and includes 1% of all bone lesions.
- 80% are diagnosed at the age of less than 30 years.
- 50% of the patients are less than 10 years old.
- The peak age is in the first decade of life.
- The multisystem type of this disease is more common in the first two years of life.
- It is slightly more common in males than females.
- More than 95% is found in Caucasians.

Source

It is probably neoplastic.
It was previously considered an immune disease.

Site

- Bone is the most common site of involvement and 77% of patients have bone involvement.
- Craniofacial bones are the most common bones involved, and cranial arch involvement is the most common site of involvement.
- Other bony involvement is the mandible, vertebral body, ribs, pelvis, and femur.
- The femur is the most common long bone involved.

- In long bones, the lesion is mostly diaphyseal or metaphyseal, and the epiphysis is almost never involved, except in very young children.
- The most common areas of extra bone are the skin, the ears, the lymph nodes, and the liver.
- The single type is twice as common as the multisystem type.

Clinical Signs

- Letterer-siwe disease: a syndrome with rapid progression of less than 3 years, the involvement of several visceral organs, every bone may be involved, most often end to death due to sepsis within 1-2 years. Tom's other: Acute diffuse-type or infant type. They typically die at less than a year. All cases are diagnosed by the age of two. Anemia, bleeding, and infection occur due to bone marrow failure. Chemotherapy may save the patient from death with systemic steroids and antibiotics.
- Hand-Schuller-christian includes the following triad:
  - Bone lesions
  - Diabetes Insipidus
  - Exophthalmos
- It is lethal at 3-10% of the cases.

Its other name is chronic diffuse type. More than 70% of the cases are diagnosed before the age of five. In addition to the symptoms mentioned, fever, anemia, hepatosplenomegaly, lymphadenopathy, and impaired liver enzymes may be observed. Chemotherapy consisting of prednisolone and vinblastine is recommended if these symptoms happend.

Bone granule ionophilization:

- The lesion is found in a few bones.
- It usually has pain.
- It may be an accidental finding.
- Local tenderness, it may have swelling.
- Fever can increase ESR.
- Nervous symptoms (collapse of the vertebral body).
- Otitis media and mastoiditis (involvement of the temporal bones)
- Tooth loss (mandibular involvement) can also be observed.

Imaging

- The typical lesion size is 1 to 2 cm.
- Lesions are usually lytic, with a definite margin, intra-medullary, and punched out lesions.
- Early phase: Aggressive permeative lesions are observed with lamellated pseudo-reaction.

- Intermediate phase: Lucent or defined margin may be scaly and endosteal scalloping. Sclerosis rim has new and thick periosteum ossification and in 5-10% of soft tissue mass.
- Delayed phase: It has peripheral sclerosis or patchy sclerosis.
- In long bones: It is a diaphyseal radiolucent lesion.

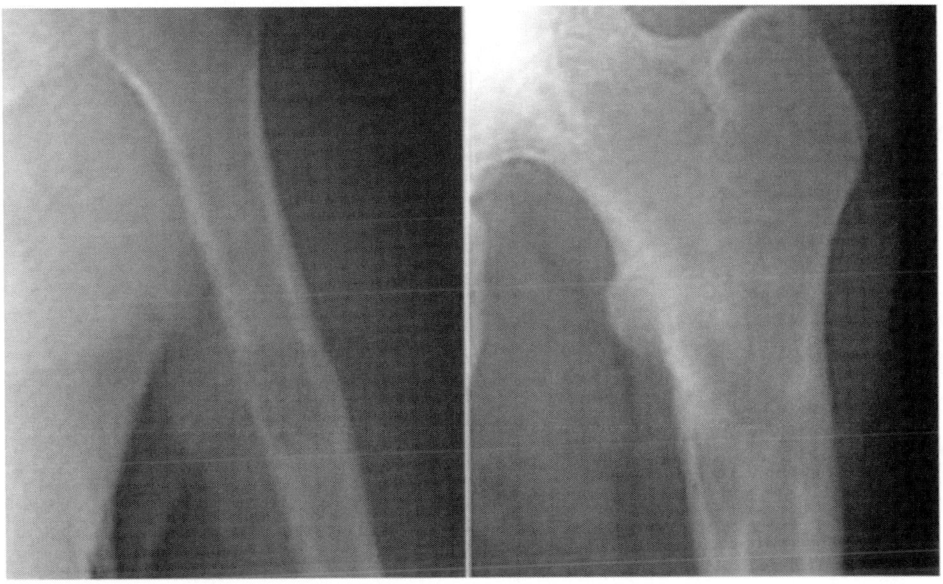

Figure 3-11. Eosinophilic granuloma. The left and right sides show the lumbosacral lesion of the Humerus and Femur, respectively.

Skull: Lytic lesion, 1 to 4 cm in size and punched out.

- Beveled margin due to uneven engagement in shallow and deep margins.
- Abscesses of the femoral head may have a central lytic lesion.
- Hole within hole view: Numerous small circular lesions which appear on the radiograph as overlapping or sticking together, resulting in one round lesion being visible over the other.
- Spine: It is shown as a vertebra plana or silver coin. With lesion repair, the height of the vertebrae can partially return. Reasons for vertebra plana are:
  - Eosinophilic granuloma: The most common etiology.
  - Lymphoma
  - Leukemia
  - Infection
  - Ewing sarcoma
  - Corner
  - ABC
- Floating teeth: It may happen because of mandibular or maxillary involvement

MRI

- It shows hidden lesions for BS radiography.
- T_1: Low to intermediate.
- T_2: Hetrograous high.
- Focal lesion surrounded by extensive edema of the bone marrow and surrounding soft tissue.
- It can look aggressive: destruction of the cortex and spread to the surrounding soft tissue can be observed.
- It has significant signal amplification with the addition of Gadolinium.

Bs

- It has a 55% increase in absorption.
- 35% is normal.
- In 10% of cases, there is a reduction in absorption.

The Potential for Malignancy

- Single lesions do not metastasize. It has a clonal origin.

Macroscopic Pathology

- Lytic foci with a distinct tan-gray border with cortical destruction.
- Tanning or yellowish foci are observed in regressive lesions or histocytes.

Microscopic Pathology

- It is made up of two types of cells: eosinophils and Langerhans cells. Only Langerhans cells are pathognomonic.
- Langerhans cells are mononulcear-histiocytic and have an oval nucleus with a distinctive oval round cytoplasm.
- Cells are positive for the S100 protein.
- Cells, left side: CD1a is positive.

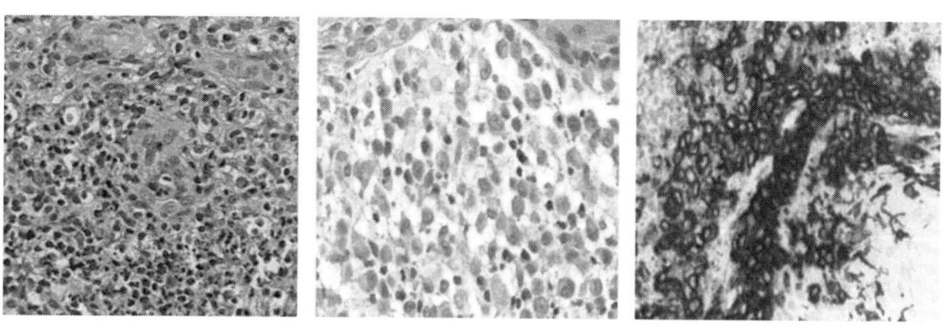

Figure 3-12. Eosinophilic granuloma. A mixture of lymphocytes, eosinophils, and Langerhans cells, Right side picture: CD1a is positive.

Treatment

- Treatment and prevention differ based on the extent of the involvement at the time of admission and also it depends on the involved organs (liver, spleen, lungs, and bone marrow).
- Individual or multifocal lesions that do not cause CNS damage can be observed or treated with steroids and then injected with steroids.
- Multisystemic patients, either with CNS damage or with involvement of dangerous internal organs such as the liver has to receive chemotherapy.
- Radiotherapy can be applied for spinal cord injuries, large or growing lesions, or if bone stabilization is needed.

Other

- LCH has to be considered in children or infants with lytic lesions in the pelvis or skull.
- The rapid progression and the disappearance of lytic lesions is characteristic of this lesion.
- If the bone scan does not increase absorption, it differentiates it from Ewing's sarcoma.
- Skeletal survey is better than a bone scan to diagnose multiple lesions, because the bone scan has a lot of false negatives.

DD

1. Single and Aggressive:
    - EWS: Patients are younger and the soft tissue mass is larger.
    - Osteomyelitis: It may differentiate before biopsy and culture.
    - Telangiectasic osteosarcoma: has a large expansile lesion with fluid-fluid surfaces.

2. Single with specified margin:
    - GCT: Expands the host by extending into the subchondral bone of the epiphysis.
    - SBC: A single-cavity lesion, with bone edema and without soft tissue component unless it is broken.
    - Brown tumor: Has other findings of hyperparathyroidism.
    - ABC: Multi-localized and expandable with fluid levels.
    - FD: The lesion is long diaphyseal, and has a frosted glass appearance.

3. Single in the recovery phase:
    - NOF: It is a lobulate that rests on the posterior cortex, as it appears to rest on the cortex.

4. Multi-focal:
    - Homogeneous osteomyelitis: The multifocal type of LCH has symptoms of involvement of other organs as well.

Chapter 4

MALIGNANT BONE TUMORS

CONVENTIONAL OSTEOSARCOMA

Definition

- It is a malignant bone tumor that malignant cells can produce osteoids or immature bone.

Epidemiology

- 10 to 25 years of age is the common age for the disease.
- M: F = 3: 2.
- It accounts for 20% of all primary malignant tumors of the bone. The second primary malignant tumor in bone.
- 30% is observed in people over 40 years. In these cases, it is secondary to Paget's disease, fibrous dysplasia, or bone infarction.
- 40% is in the distal femur.
- The next most common sites are the proximal tibia and proximal humerus.
- 90% is metaphysis.

Clinical Signs

- Ambiguous pain is the most common complaint, especially at night.
- Almost all patients have progressive pain (patients with low-grade superficial osteosarcoma may complain of swelling).
- Night pain occurs in only 25% of patients.
- The pain lasts from several weeks to several months.
- The average delay from the onset of symptoms to diagnosis is 15 weeks. 6 weeks is because of patients delay to visit a doctor and 9 weeks is related to delay in patient diagnostic process.

- The delay in the diagnostic process is related to the faults in requesting and repeating the radiograph from the patient.

Another reason for the delay in diagnosing is the good general condition of osteosarcoma patients which may cause to underestimate the disease.

- A palpable mass develops after the pain intensifies.
- The skin is warm and has prominent arteries.
- The palpable mass is associated with a decrease in the ROM of the adjacent joint.
- Some patients have weight loss at the time of diagnosis, accompanied by the spread of the disease to other organs and is mostly pulmonary metastasis.
- Increased LDH and ALP can be observed. Some studies have shown that increasing these two laboratory tests is associated with poor prognosis. Alkaline phosphatase monitors are useful in assessing the response to chemotherapy. Local recurrence or metastasis may occur if the decreased alkaline phosphatase increases again after treatment.
- Pathological fractures is observed in 20% of the cases.

Imaging

- It has a variable appearance (amorphous or cloudy appearance) depending on the value of bone matrix.
- The site of the tumor is metaphysis: 10% is diaphyseal, and 1% epiphyseal.
- It is typically a mixed radiograph of sclerosis and lucent, but can be completely lytic or sclerotic.
- It has a wide transitional zone with an aggressive view (destruction of the cortex and soft tissue component).
- Aggressive periosteal reactions like disorganized, sunburst, or hair on end are common like the Cadman triangle. Cadman Triangle is an insufficient attempt by Periost to limit the tumor. It can be observed in infection as well.

Staging

- CT and MRI are useful for preoperative planning to find the extent of bone involvement. T_1 coronal cut of the entire length of the involved bone is used to determine the extent of tumor involvement within the bone, and T_2 axial cut to determine the involvement of extraosseous structures. Bone metastasis greater than 2 mm is observed in bone MRI.
- Bone scans are used to find bone metastasis.
- CT scan of the lungs is to detect lung metastasis. Pulmonary metastasis of three to seven millimeters is observed on a CT scan. A Spiral CT scan is better in this regard. Pulmonary metastasis of one centimeter or more is observed on chest radiographs.

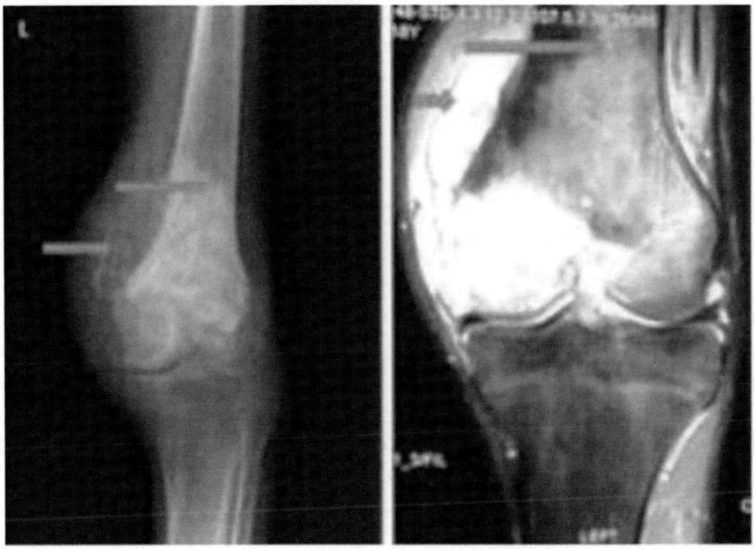

Figure 4-1. Osteosarcoma. Left: Radiography of the anterior-posterior. Radiopaque lesion with indistinct margin and corroded cortex in the distal metaphysis and epiphysis of the femur. The up and down arrows represent the soft tissue component and the intra-medullary spread of the tumor, respectively. Right: T2 coronary MRI with fat suppressor. The up and down arrows represent the soft tissue component and the intra-medullary spread of the tumor.

Macroscopic Pathology

- A mixture of bony and non-bony areas, heterogeneous in color, consistency.
- Areas of intense bone are white to yellowish in color.
- Non-bony areas are tanned, fleshy or cartilaginous.

Microscopic Pathology

- It has two basic components: sarcomatous tumor cells and extracellular matrix.
- Finding the production of bone matrix by tumor sarcomatous cells is essential for diagnosis.
- Depending on the type of dominant matrix, it is divided into three types: osteoblastic, chondroblastic and fibroblastic.

Treatment

Preoperative chemotherapy: Preoperative chemotherapy controls possible metastasis sooner, can reduce tumor volume and facilitate surgery, and knowing the tumor's response to chemotherapy helps to determine the prognosis. If the tumor has no response to chemotherapy, stopping preoperative surgery and earlier surgery will not help to survive. There is no change in prognosis whether the entire dose of chemotherapy is given after surgery or part of it is given before and part of it after surgery.

The existence of more than 90% necrosis following initial chemotherapy is considered a good prognosis. Some state this as 98%. Changing the chemotherapy regimen in those with less than 90% necrosis has not been shown to have a better outcome for patients.

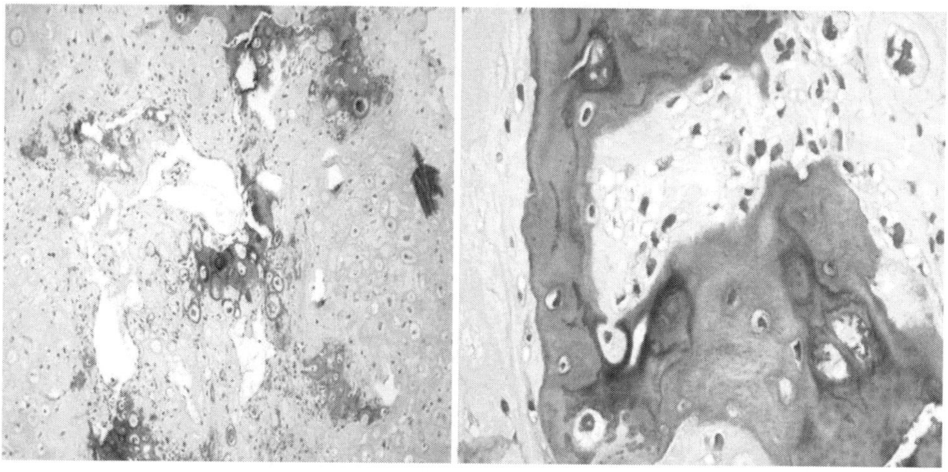

Figure 4-2. Conventional osteosarcoma: Osteoids are found as nets around anaplastic tumor cells.

The existence of multidrug resistance (MDR) gene resistant to chemotherapy drugs pumps the drugs out of the cell by cancer cells. These genes are present in 25% of primary tumors and 50% of metastasis. About twenty to forty percent of osteosarcomas do not respond to treatment. It is not yet clear whether imaging with laboratory findings will help identify this subgroup or not.

- If a large margin is obtained during surgery, the survival of patients with organ retention is no different from amputation.

Sub

- Lung metastasis can be due to pneumothorax necrosis of the pleural surface.
- Pulmonary metastasis with an osteoid matrix has a worse prognosis.
- Osteosarcoma is not associated with lymphadenopathy. If lytic, sclerotic lesions on radiograph were associated with lymphadenopathy, osteomyelitis has to be considered more than osteosarcoma.

Differential Diagnosis of Lytic Type

- Infection: In this case, the soft tissue component is smaller and has a history of infection. It has a sinus tract.
- Fracture: Has a history of trauma. The component has no soft texture. Follow-up is in the process of improving.

Dense Type Differential Diagnosis

- Condor sarcoma: Most of the axillary skeleton is involved.
- Occipital myositis: Calcification is more mature in the lesion environment, unlike osteosarcoma, which has a soft tissue component in most environments.
- Cortical desmoid: It is observed only in the posterior metaphyseal condyle of the femoral condyle.

TYPES OF OSTEO SARCOMA

Primitive

- Conventional
- Telangiectatic
- Parosteal
- High load surface
- Intramedullary upward
- Small cell
- Secondary: will be described.

TELANGIECTATIC OSTEOSARCOMA

Definition

- It is a malignant ossification tumor where hyperemic tumors are surrounded by septa containing neoplastic sarcomatous cells.

Epidemiology

- 2F = M.
- Common age: 10 to 25 years.
- Less than 5% of osteosarcomas.

Common Site

- The site resembles the usual type of osteosarcoma, both inside the bone and skeleton.
- 10% is completely diaphysis.

Clinical Signs

- Pain: The pain has lasted for several weeks to several months.
- Pain is associated with swelling and limited movement.
- Pathological fractures are observed in 25%.

Radiography

- Fully lytic geographical lesion with permeative growth view

- It often dilates the bone and destroys the cortex, yet the periosteal reaction is small and has an onion skin appearance.
- The radiological appearance is more of Ewing's sarcoma rather than osteosarcoma.
- The radiological appearance can be deceptive, resembling a benign lesion like a bone aneurysmal cyst.
- Cortex rupture is observed in 89% of MRIs.
- Fluid-fluid levels and bag of blood can be observed on CT and MRI.
- Donut sign: It is observed on a bone scan. It has an increased uptake in margins unlike the center of the lesion.

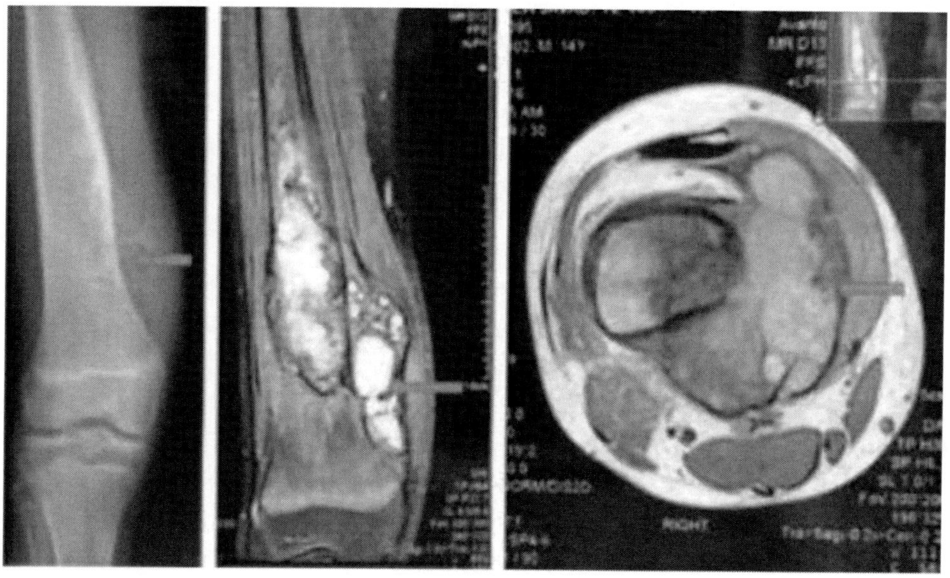

Figure 4-3. Telangiectasic osteosarcoma in a 14-year-old teenager. Left: plain radiograph. Radiocentric lesion with the destruction of the medial metaphyseal cortex of the distal femur. The arrow shows the component of the lesion. Middle and right: T2 coronary MRI with fat suppress and axial T1. The arrows show the large soft tissue component of the tumor.

Malignancy Potential

- Similar to 65% modular type, it has 5-year survival.

Macroscopic Pathology

- It is very hemorrhagic and looks like a bag of blood.
- Includes necrosis and cystic cavities.
- The sarcomatosis meaty component is usually absent or very small.
- Similar to ABC.

Microscopic Pathology

- In is observed a lot in sarcomatous tumor septa, severe atypical pleomorphism.
- Sometimes it does not have a septum and sarcomatous cells float in the blood.
- The covering layer of cysts is tumor cells and does not have a true endothelial layer.
- Osteogenesis is negligible.

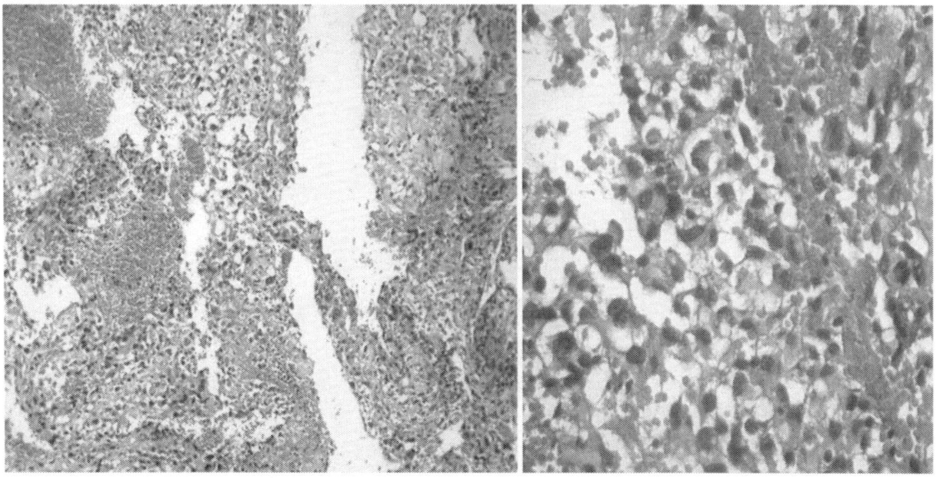

Figure 4-4. Telangiectatic osteosarcoma: The covering layer of cysts is tumor cells and does not have a true endothelial layer.

Other

- Associated with Paget and retinoblastoma.

DD

- ABC: Unlike ABC, osteosarcoma has the following features:
- It destroys the cortex and soft tissue mass.
- Mineralized matrix is best observed at the margin of the lesion on CT.
- Solid tissue is found around cystic spaces.
- GCT: It is the epiphysis. It has no bone matrix.

Osteomyelitis: There is less bleeding and fluid levels.
FD: The frosted glass view is observed without damaging the cortex.

Parosteal Osteosarcoma

Definition

- It is a low-grade ossifying sarcoma where the bone surface is exophytic without lifting the periosteum.
- It contains components with spindle cells and tumor bone trabeculae.
- It attacks the bone medulla only in the final stages.

Epidemiology

- Normally, it is observed after skeletal puberty.
- The peak age is in the third and fourth decades, 50% are over 30 years of age.

- F> M.

It consists of 3% of osteosarcomas.

Site

- 80% are observed in the posterior femoral shaft above the popliteal space.
- The proximal tibia is the next most common site, observed entirely in the metaphysis and shaft.
- It has also been reported in the proximal humerus and other long bones.
- Related to previous radiotherapy.

Signs

- Painless Stiff swelling with no movement is a common symptom.
- In the history of the patient, there may be a history of a biopsy or attempts for surgery a lesion that is thought to be benign.
- If the lesion is in the posterior distal femor, it is hard to bend the knee.

Imaging

- The tumor grows on the surface of the bone and attaches to it with a broad base.
- It is densely mineralized and has a lobulated margin.
- There is a cauliflower or fungal shaped on the surface view of the bone that looks to be attached to the host bone, but there is space between the tumor and the host bone.
- There is no new periosteal ossification because of the tumor not being lifted by the tumor.
- The tumor is sometimes wrapped around the bone. It can have cartilaginous gaps. It has up to 25% invasion of bone marrow and soft tissue. This condition is observed in very late stages.
- A CT scan may help to differentiate this tumor from ossifican myositis or osteo chondroma.
- In ossifican myositis, ossification is more pronounced around the peripheral than the center. This is in contrast to parosteal osteosarcoma.
- In osteochondroma, the medullary canal of the bone is along the medullary canal of the tumor.

Malignancy Potential

- Prognosis is better than conventional type.
- Consequence has a bad outcome of recurrence if the lesion is dedifferentiated. It rarely loses its differentiation in tumors with recurrent lesions.

Macroscopic Pathology

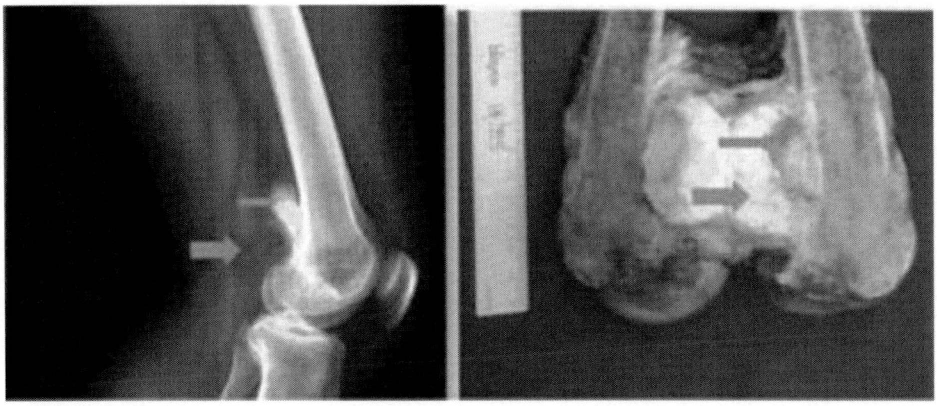

Figure 4-5. Parosteal osteosarcoma. Left: plain radiograph and right side distal femoral specimen. The upper arrows show the bony part of the lesion and the lower ones the cartilaginous part of the tumor. Unlike ossifican myositis, calcification is more severe in the center than in the peripheral.

Microscopic Pathology

- It is composed of slightly atypical spindle cells that form slightly atypical bone trabeculae.

Treatment

- Extensive surgical resection of the tumor.
- Chemotherapy is not indicated unless the tumor has a high grade.

Differential Diagnosis

- Myositis ossificans: It is completely separate from the bone and has no adhesions. In myositis ossificans, ossification is more mature in the peripheral, while in parosteal osteosarcoma, it is more intense at the center of ossification.
- Osteochondroma: The bone marrow extends along the tumor.
- Prosthetic osteosarcoma: It is rarer, more common in the tibia, more likely to have a sunburst-type periosteal reaction, younger patients.
- Intraosseous parosteal lipoma: The component has fat.
- Nora lesion: It is observed on the hands and feet. It is also called bizarre parosteal BPOP osteochondromatous proliferous.

Other

- It originates from the outer layer of the periosteum and no periosteal reaction is observed.
- CT and MRI show that the lesion is not along the modular canal of the bone, so it is not exostosis.
- About 25% to 30% have a cartilaginous cap.
- The dedifferentiated type of this tumor has a worse prognosis similar to the prognosis of periosteal osteosarcoma.

- Needle biopsy is useless in determining the grade of the tumor because the tumor has heterogeneous areas.

Periosteal Osteosarcoma

Definition

- A low- to moderate-grade bone marrow sarcoma with a predominantly cartilaginous distinction found on the surface of the pediatrics bone.

Epidemiology

- It is very rare.
- Peak age is in the second decade. Patients are slightly older than conventional osteosarcoma.

Source

- It originates from the inner layer of the periosteum. It has a lot of cartilaginous matrices.

Site

- Lower limbs. The tibia and then the femur are the most common bones involved.
- In long bones, it is more diaphyseal than metaphyseal.

Clinical Signs

- Swelling with or without pain for weeks to months is a common symptom.
- At first, it can be a painless lump.
- Gradually progresses to pain and tenderness.
- 25% have pathological fractures.

Imaging

- Most often, it is observed as a spindle-shaped mass, mostly radiolucent located on the surface of a long bone.
- The sunburst, Cadman triangle and smooth bone mass can occur.

- Scalloping of the external cortex is observed.
- It does not typically enter the modular canal.
- The subperiosteal site of the tumor is observed by a CT scan or MRI.

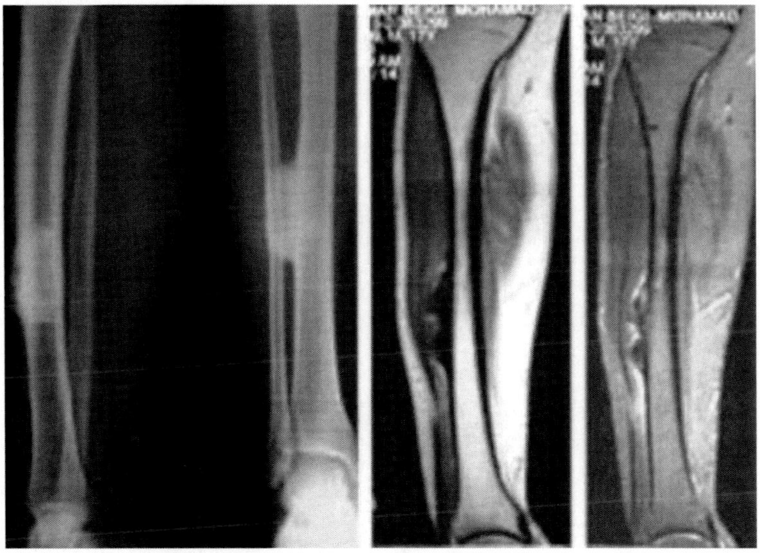

Figure 4-6. Periosteal osteosarcoma in the tibial diaphysis. Left: A plain radiograph shows radiopaque attached to the bone cortex. Middle and right: T1 and T2 coronary MRI with a fat suppressor, respectively. In both views, due to the presence of an abundant calcification, a low signal lesion can be observed. It can also be observed that the lesion did not involve the medulla.

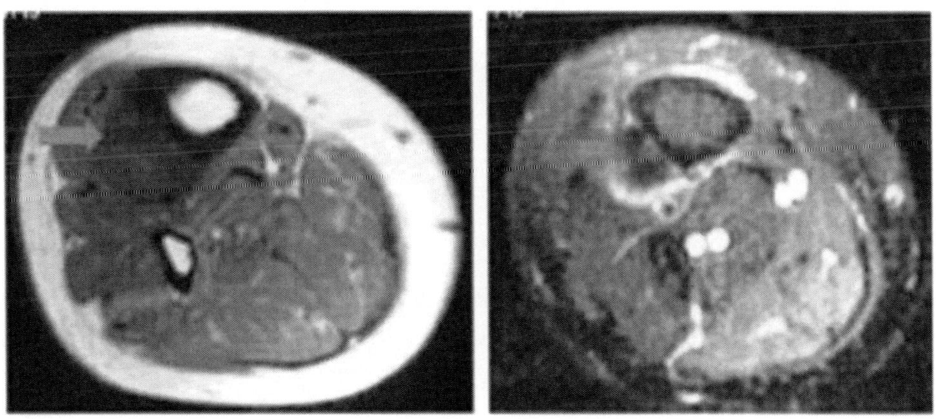

Figure 4-7. Periosteal osteosarcoma. Left and right: T1 and T2 MRI with fat suppress. The arrows show a tumor observed as a low signal in both views due to the presence of abundant calcification. It is well observed in axial cuts that did not involve a medullary tumor.

Malignancy Potential

- It is better than conventional type and worse than parosteal type.

Macroscopic Pathology

- It is a spindle-shaped tumor with a distinct margin of the surrounding bone.
- Periosteal elevation and spikes due to reactive periosteal ossification may be observed.
- Cartilage within the tumor is common.
- May have a lobulated appearance.

Microscopic Pathology

- It has a predominantly cartilaginous appearance.

The apparent cartilaginous component of the atypical cell is equivalent to chondrosarcoma grade 2 to 3.

- In the area between the cartilage lobules, sarcomatous cells with osteoid production are observed.

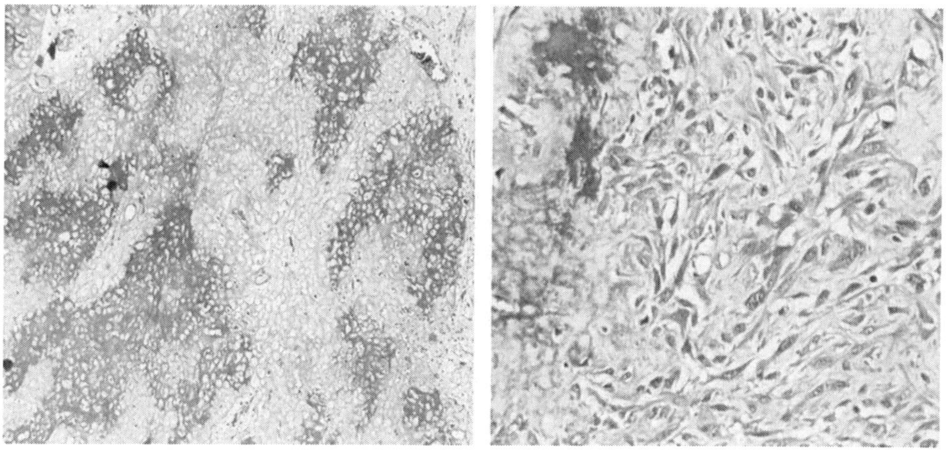

Figure4-8. Periosteal osteosarcoma.

Treatment

- Tumor removal with a wide margin is the standard treatment for this tumor.
- Chemotherapy is used for patients, although its benefits are questionable.
- Chemotherapy is used for patients whose tumor contains dedifferentiated or high-grade areas.

DD

- Prostate Chondroma/Chondrosarcoma: It may pose compressive erosion on the bone and the cartilaginous matrix. Periosteal chondroma is involved in 50% of the proximal humerus and then the small bones of the hand are involved. The radiographic view of the lesion is a central depression with prominent edges.
- High-grade superficial osteosarcoma: Radiography is hard for differentiation.
- Parosteal osteosarcoma: The prevalence is higher. It is difficult to differentiate from each other.
- Osteochondroma: The cortex and bone marrow continue in the tumor.

- Osteoid Osteoma: It has nidus. It has no soft texture component.
- Osteomyelitis: Periosteal involvement is observed around the bone and not as a focal mass.

High-Grade Superficial Osteosarcoma

Definition

- High-grade osteosarcoma that develops on the surface of the bone and does not involve the modular canal.

Epidemiology

- It is very rare. It is the rarest type of osteosarcoma.
- It is observed in adolescents and young adults.
- It is more common in males.

Site

- It originates from the surface of the long bone in the metaphyseal region.
- Long bones (femur, tibia, humerus and fibula) are more involved.
- The distal femur and proximal humerus are the most common areas involved.

Clinical Signs

- Pain and swelling are the most common complaints.
- The duration of symptoms varies from a few months to several years.

Imaging

- It is observed as a mineralized mass on the bone surface.
- Radiographs show an invasive lesion with an indistinct margin at the bone surface.
- Unlike the parosteal type, medullary canal involvement is observed very early in the disease.
- hypercellularity, mitosis, and nuclear pleomorphism is observed in the pathology of this tumor (like conventional type)
- The degree of mineralization varies and is generally similar to conventional type mineralization.

- Similar to the prosthetic type, the periosteal reaction can be observed as a cadmium triangle.

Intra-Medullary Osteosarcoma of the Lower Grade

- It has a slow head and a relatively benign appearance on radiography.
- In some patients, radiographically and histologically, it may not be mistaken for osteoblastoma or fibrous dysplasia.
- If left untreated, it may perforate the cortex at a very late stage.
- M = F
- They are older than conventional osteosarcoma. The peak age is in the third decade, but cases of the disease have been observed in people over 50 years of age.
- The femur is the most common bone involved. It is then observed in the tibia.
- Sclerosis is more.
- Prognosis is better, but recurrence can be high grade.
- It is composed of slightly atypical spindle cells that make slightly atypical bony trabeculae.

Small Cell Osteosarcoma

- Its epidemiology is similar to osteosarcoma.
- It is similar to Ewing's sarcoma or lymphoma. It is composed of small blue cells.
- To differentiate it with Ewing's sarcoma, it may need cytogenetics or immunohistochemical staining.
- It is often lytic and has a permeative appearance, but also has small areas of osteoids.
- It tends to spread in the bone shaft.
- The prognosis is slightly worse than the usual type of osteosarcoma.
- Slightly more common in females.

SECONDARY

Epidemiology

- About half of all osteosarcoma cases are in people over the age of 50.
- The most common causes of Paget's disease are the previous radiotherapy.

Paget's Disease

- Between 1 to 0% of patients with Paget's disease develop osteosarcoma, depending on the extent of the involvement.
- 50-60% of sarcomas form on the surface of osteosarcoma.
- Osteotic type is more likely to be observed in Paget type than monostotic.
- It is observed in the sixth to eighth decades.
- The pelvis is the most common site of involvement.

- The prognosis is poor and less than 15% have a long life.

Radiotherapy

- It is observed in 1% of patients who have the history of receiving more than 2,500 radiotherapy.
- It is found in unusual areas like the skull, spine, clavicle, ribs, scapula, and pelvis.
- It accounts for 50-60% of radiation sarcomas. Fibrosarcoma and MFH may be observed too.
- Children receiving radiotherapy are at higher risk.
- The average latency is 10 to 15 years.
- Increasing radiation dose is directly related to increasing risk of the disease.

Other Underlying Causes of Secondary Osteosarcoma

- Fibrous dysplasia
- Osteogeneis Imperfecta
- Hardware
- Chronic osteomyelitis
- Osteochondroma
- Melorheostosis
- Bone infarct

Bad Prognosis in OS

- Age and gender are ineffective.
- Higher Stage. It is the most important prognostic factor.
- Non-pulmonary metastasis.
- Skip metastasis.
- High grade.
- Larger tumor size.
- Proximal tumor.
- It is secondary to Paget.
- Secondary to radiotherapy. In this case, the tumor site has an effective role, like osteosarcoma, secondary to radiotherapy in the peripheral areas of the limb has a prognosis, similar to primary grade high-grade osteosarcoma.
- Rapid recurrence occurs after treatment.
- Pulmonary nodules more than 8.
- Pulmonary nodules larger than 3 cm
- Non-surgical resection of pulmonary nodules.
- Pulmonary nodules that make osteoids.

Good Prognosis in OS

- If 90% of the tumor necrosis due to preoperative chemotherapy.

Miscellaneous in the Case of Conventional Osteosarcoma

- The presence of interferon α / β receptor is a good prognostic factor in osteosarcoma.

Chemotherapy

- The goals are:
- Elimination of metastasis (micro-and-macro metastasis)
- Make LSS (limb Salvage Surgery) possible.
- Surgery will be 3-4 weeks after pre-operative chemotherapy
- 2 weeks from the operation is the start of postoperative chemotherapy provided that the patient's wound has healed.
- If less than 90% of the tumor necrosis is due to preoperative chemotherapy, the same preoperative drugs can be repeated.
- Necrosis of more than 90% is associated with a very good prognosis.
- If> 90% of the cells become necrotic, increasing the dose does not change the patient's survival by changing chemotherapy medicines.

Radiotherapy

- Because of radiation resistance, radiotherapy has only a palliative role.

Surgery

- The base of treatment is surgery (both the primary tumor and its metastasis).
- The current recommendation for metastasis is to resect them as much as possible.
- Limb salvage can be done for more than 85% of peripheral skeletal osteosarcoma. Proper margin for bone is two to five centimeters beyond the bone involvement in the MRI and five to ten millimeters beyond the soft tissue component of the tumor. The foraminal margin is better than fat margin. In boys over the age of twelve and in girls over the age of ten, we select the length of the prosthesis or allograft to regenerate the limbs up to two centimeters longer to stop the growth of the two limbs. In children younger than the above, after completing chemotherapy, treatment has to be considered to lift the limb or use an elongated prosthesis.
- Amputation is the gold standard of local disease control and provides the most functional reconstruction for sports purposes. Indications for amputation in osteosarcoma include young children, large masses of soft tissue involving the neurovascular, progression of osteosarcoma during preoperative chemotherapy, local recurrence following surgery, and displaced pathologic fractures. In the upper extremities, every effort has to be made to maintain the function of the hand because the function of the hand is not comparable to the best prosthesis.

For Further Reading

- AAOS 2009/ Vol 17, No:8.

- Small cell Osteosarcoma Cytopathologic Characterisitis and Differential Diagnosis, Justin A Bishop MD, Chung H Shum MD, PhD, Sheila Sheth MD, Paul E.Wakely Jr MD, Syed Z. Ali MD. Am J Clin Pathol 2010; 133:756-761.

Conventional Chondrosarcoma

Definition

- It is a malignant tumor of the cartilage in which the matrix created is exponentially chondroid.

Epidemiology

- It accounts for 90% of primary malignant bone tumors.
- Incidence is ½ comparing osteosarcoma.
- It has a second prevalence in primary bone sarcomas.
- The commonest age is between 40 and 60 years for the primary type, and between 25 and 45 years for the secondary type.
- Slightly more common in males than females.
- According to some authors, the prevalence is equal in both sexes.
- Racial superiority is not observed.
- 20 to 27% of all primary bone sarcomas.
- It accounts for 80-90% of all chondrosarcomas.

Source

- It is typically low grade. Malignant contains hyaline cartilage.

Primary type: not created on another lesion.

Secondary type: Come from other lesions like osteochondroma (most common), enchondroma, periosteal chondroma, Paget, radiation therapy (see the end of the season)

Site

- The pelvis, ribs, femur, humerus, scapula, and sternum are the most common sites involved.
- The pelvis and ribs, each account for 20% of the disease and are the most common areas involved.
- The ilium is the most common single bone involved.
- It is rare in hands, feet, craniofacial and spine.

- In the hand, although rare, it is the most common primary bone cancer.
- It is metadiaphyseal.
- It is much more common in the long bones in the proximal than distal.
- The axial skeleton is involved more than the appendix.

Clinical Signs

- Most of the patients report increasing pain.
- Local swelling can be observed because of bone dilation or due to the spread of the tumor into the soft tissue.
- Symptoms usually last for several months, yet they may last for years.
- Pain is important in the absence of pathological fractures and helps to differentiate chondrosarcoma from enchondroma.
- Pain at rest and nocturnal pain are symptoms making the patient visit the hospital.
- The pain is vague and may be intermittent.
- Pain is especially important in a lesion without previous pain.
- Restriction of joint movement can be observed in near bone terminal tumors.
- Pathological fractures are observed in 3 to 17%.

Imaging

- Lytic view with opacity points (Arcs & Ring) with more or less uniform distribution.
- The pattern of calcification is dotted comma-shaped or popcorn.
- Aggressive appearance with bone destruction, cortical erosion, periosteal reaction, and rarely soft tissue component helps to differentiate it from the enchondroma.
- It is usually larger than 4 cm.
- Zone of transition is variable.
- Smooth Endosteal scalloping and thickened cortex is a sign of slow tumor growth.
- The periosteal reaction can be several layers in parallel and foggy form (slow growth).
- The periosteal reaction is more aggressive and the rupture of the cortex is observed in more aggressive types.

CT

- It is better than MRI in showing cartilage matrix and endosteal scalloping or cortical destruction.
- It shows the destruction of surrounding bone by cartilage matrix.
- The site of the tumor has to be considered in the interpretation of cortical destruction, as in the case of destruction of the cortex by a cartilaginous tumor, it can be considered benign. However, in the pelvis and proximal limb the same amount of destruction (more than two-thirds of cortical thickness) in invasive types.

CT

- It is better than MRI in showing cartilage matrix and endosteal scalloping or cortical destruction.
- It shows the destruction of surrounding bone by a cartilaginous matrix.
- The site of the tumor has to be considered in the interpretation of cortical destruction as in the case of destruction of the cortex by a cartilaginous tumor it can be considered benign, but in the pelvis and proximal limb the same amount of destruction (more than two-thirds of the cortex thickness) is a sign of malignancy.

MRI

- In T2 view, it is very clear because of the high water content in the hyaline cartilage inside the tumor.
- Secondary chondrosarcoma has to be considered if the size of the cartilaginous cap in adult osteochondroma is greater than 2 cm.
- It has a lobulated growth view.

BS

- Increased heterogeneity absorption is greater than the iliac crest anterior.

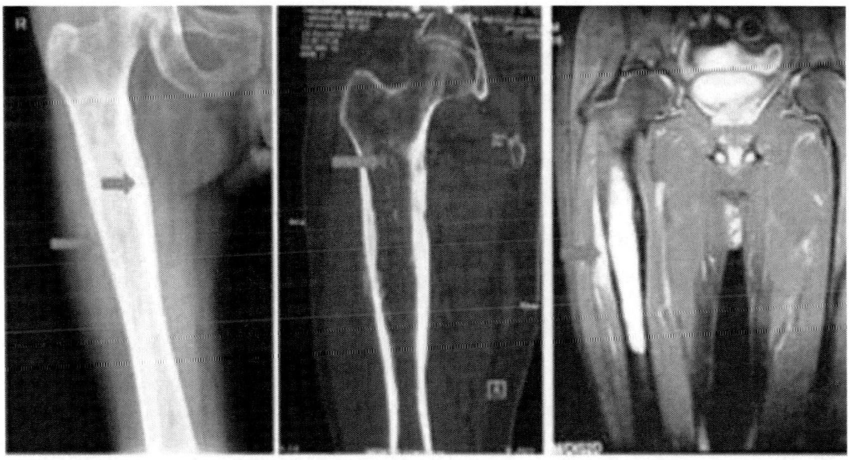

Figure 4-9. Right thigh conventional chondrosarcoma. Left: plain radiograph. The upper arrow shows the thickening of the cortex and the bottom arrow shows the soft tissue component. Middle: CT scan. The arrow indicates chondroid calcification. Right: Coronary MRI. The arrow represents the soft tissue component.

Malignancy Potential

- High-grade varieties have a 5% recurrence with a 5-year survival.
- The most significant predictor of local recurrence and metastasis is tumor grade.
- Grading is associated with the clinical behavior of the tumor.

Macroscopic Pathology

- It has a lobulated structure.
- It has translucent hyaline nodules that are similar to normal cartilage.

- Ivory areas are a sign of ossification.
- Fragile and hemorrhagic gray tissue with a fleshy appearance is a sign of a high-grade tumor.

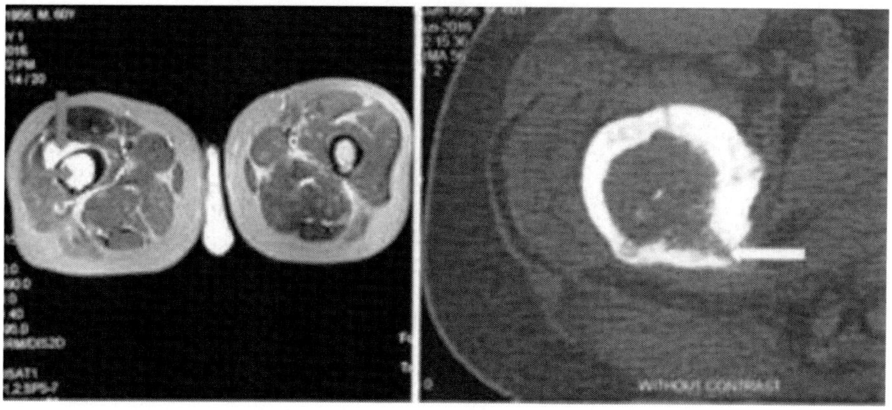

Figure 4-10. Conventional right thigh chondrosarcoma. Left: MRI T2 fat suppress. The arrows show the component inside and outside the bone of the tumor, observed in this view with a high signal. Right: CT scan of the axial cut. The arrow indicates a ruptured cortex.

Microscopic Pathology

- It is composed of malignant cells with abundant cartilage matrix.
- Tumors are uniformly cartilaginous.
- The presence of even a small amount of osteoids shows the diagnosis of chondroblastic osteosarcoma.
- Tumor cells, like normal chondrocytes are located inside lacunae in the hyaline cartilage matrix.
- The progressive cartilaginous margin of the chondrosarcoma invades the bony trabeculae
- Areas of myxoid and calcification may be observed.
- Tumor lobules vary from less than 1 mm to a few millimeters.

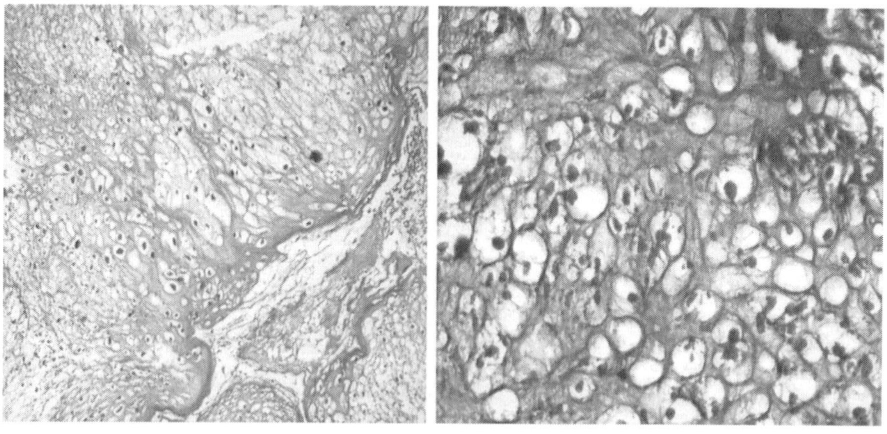

Figure 4-11. Chondrosarcoma: It is composed of malignant cells with abundant cartilage matrix. Tumor cells, like normal chondrocytes, are located inside lacunae in the hyaline cartilage matrix.

Treatment

- The preferred treatment is wide resection. However, depending on the grade, the treatment can change.
- Low grade: Extensive curettage with thermal ablation/chemical + graft or cement. This treatment is only considered for low-grade tumors limited to a sufficient medullary canal.
- Tumors with soft tissue spread has to be treated like high-grade tumors.
- High grade: wide excision with chemotherapy and radiotherapy.
- Radiotherapy is used if the tumor is not surgical.
- Chemotherapy is used for the mesenchymal and dedifferentiated types.
- 5-year survival.
  - Grade 1: 90%.
  - Grade 2: 81%.
  - Grade 3: 29%.
- Metastasis
  - Grade 1: NA
  - Grade 2: 10%.
  - Grade 3: 60%.
- As the cartilage is avascular, tumor cells are easily implanted in the surrounding tissue, and recurrence is high after infection during surgery.
- For lesions in dilated bones, extensive early resection without biopsy may be indicated to reduce the risk of infection.

DD

- Enchondroma: No invasive symptoms (cortex rupture, endoscopic scalloping, soft tissue component of the periosteal reaction). Enchondroma is rare in the pelvis, ribs, sternum, and scapula.
- Osteosarcoma: Has an osteoid matrix.
- Osifican myositis: It is not attached to the bone, more densely mineralized in the lesion environment than its center.

Osteonecrosis with secondary sarcoma: Secondary calcification: Calcification is more pronounced in the environment.

Other

- Grade 2 and 1 have similar clinical behavior.
- Synovial chondromatosis, Oliver's disease, periosteal chondroma, or hand enchondroma, atypia, and hypercellularity may exist but still benign, but a pathological appearance in a pelvic lesion showing radiography of the cortex suggests a diagnosis of chondrosarcoma, all of them have to be used in conjunction with the clinical and radiological model to achieve the diagnosis.

TYPES OF CHONDROSARCOMA PRIMERS

Conventional

- It is the most common subgroup.
- It grows slowly.

Clear Cell

M: F = 2 · 4

- It is very rare. It covers 2% of the cases.
- A radiolucent lesion of the end of the bone with a sclerotic rim (similar to chondroblastoma).
- It can be radiolucent or highly mineralized.
- The maximum prevalence is in the third and fourth decades.
- The femoral head (45%), the humerus and the pelvis are the most common sites of involvement, respectively.
- Chondrosarcoma is considered low-grade.
- The patient usually presents with pain. It may be painful for years due to slow growth.
- It is composed of round cells with abundant clear cytoplasm and distinct cell margins in the cartilaginous matrix.
- Giant cells are multinucleated.
- Complete treatment is en bloc resection. Marginal resection usually leads to recurrence.
- The overall recurrence is 20%. The average recurrence time is 1.7 years and the metastasis time is 8 years after diagnosis.
- Chemotherapy is effective in increasing life expectancy.

Juxta Cortical

- It is also called periosteal chondrosarcoma.
- It is slightly more common than clear cell.
- The most common age is the third and fourth decade.

M = F

- It is a type of Conventional Chondrosarcoma found on the surface of the bone and is extramedullary.
- The diaphysis or metaphyseal surface of long bones, such as the femur and tibia, is involved.

- On CT and MRI, the surfaces are lifted by the periosteum and covered deep by the bone cortex.
- The cortex is usually observed.
- It can have a multilayer periosteal reaction.
- It is usually larger than five centimeters.
- It is similar to the periosteal osteochondroma and the periosteal osteosarcoma.

Mesenchymal: 3%

- It is very rare. It involves 3% of the cases. In terms of prevalence, it is the boundary between clear cell and juxta cortical.
- M = F.
- The most common age is 20 to 30 years.
- The lower limbs, pelvis, spine and upper and lower jaw are common sites of involvement.
- Involvement of the central nervous system by tumor invasion of the skull or spine is a characteristic of this type.
- Involvement of the central nervous system by tumor invasion of the skull or spine is its characteristic.
- It is a lytic lesion with a soft tissue component.
- In half of the cases, the soft tissue component is observed.
- It is a high-grade chondrosarcoma.
- It has small round blue cells that appear to be normal along with the cartilaginous islands.
- Its pathological appearance is similar to hemangiomas with deer-like vessels.
- The five-year lifespan is less than 50%. Chemotherapy is especially helpful if it looks like Ewing's sarcoma under a microscope and increases the length.

Dedifferentiated

- It accounts for 11% of the cases.
- It includes a high-grade sarcoma (most commonly osteosarcoma, then fibrosarcoma and MFH) rejecting the presence of a typical low-grade chondrosarcoma.
- It is called chondrosarcoma with grade 1 or 2 becoming a high-grade sarcoma.
- The age is often over 50 years. The average age is about 60 years.
- Common areas of conflict are similar to the conventional type.
- Recent changes in pain pattern or increase in previous mass size is in favor of this diagnosis.
- On radiography, it appears as an aggressive radiolucent region adjacent to typical chondrosarcoma.
- Pathological fractures are observed up to 50%.
- It has the worst prognosis.

- In pathology, it has at least two components.
    - Well-differentiated cartilage lesion.
    - High-grade sarcoma.
        - Sudden histological deformation happens between the two pathological components of the tumor.
        - Dedifferentiation can also be observed in low-grade intramedullary osteosarcoma, parosteal osteosarcoma, liposarcoma, and GCT.

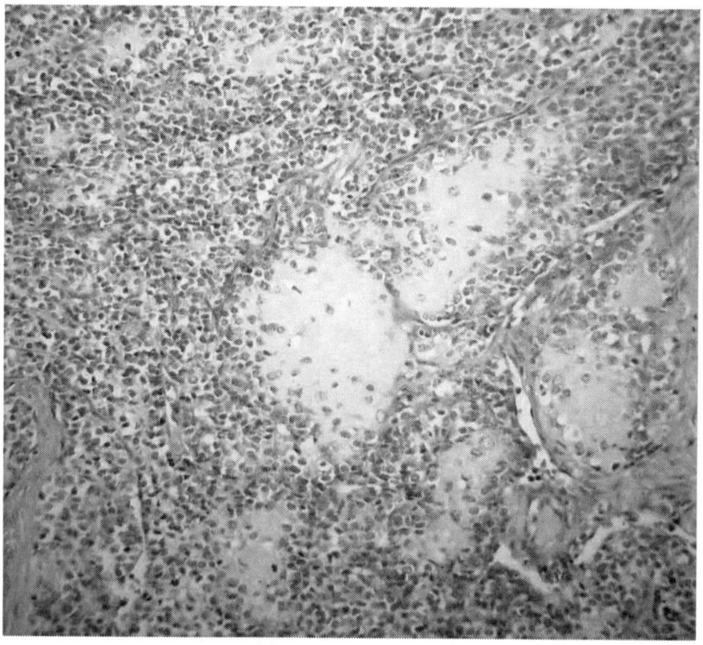

Figure 4-12. Mesenchymal chondrosarcoma: Biphasic pattern, composed of cellular round blue cells with islands of well differentiated hyalin cartilage.

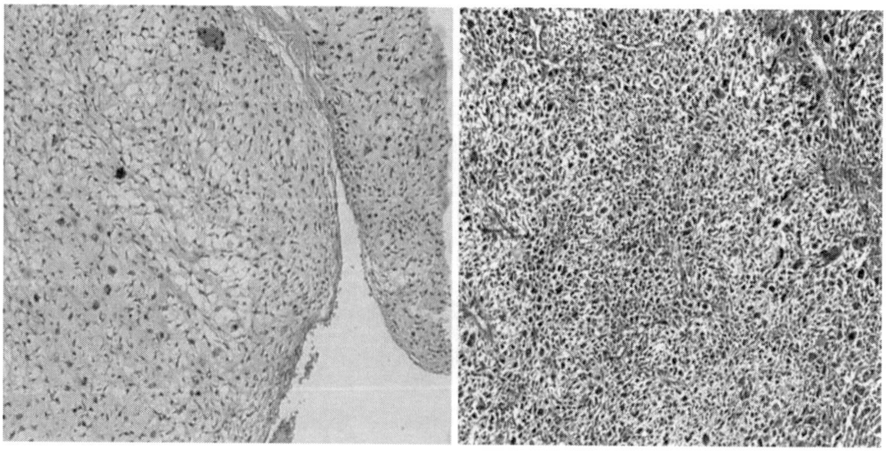

Figure 4-13. Dedifferentiated ChondroSarcoma: High-grade sarcoma (right image) is observed adjacent to a typical lower-grade chondrosarcoma (left image).

Extraosseous: % 2

- It accounts for 11% of the cases and is rare in people under 40 years of age.
- 80% is in the lower extremities.
- The appearance of the tumor is low-grade lobulated calcification.
- It can be observed in the context of the following conditions.
- Enchondroma.
- Osteochondroma.
- Irradiated bone.
- Periosteal chondroma.
- Paget disease.
- Synovial chondromatosis.
- Fibrous dysplasia.
- Chonodromyxoid fibroma.
- Chondroblastoma.

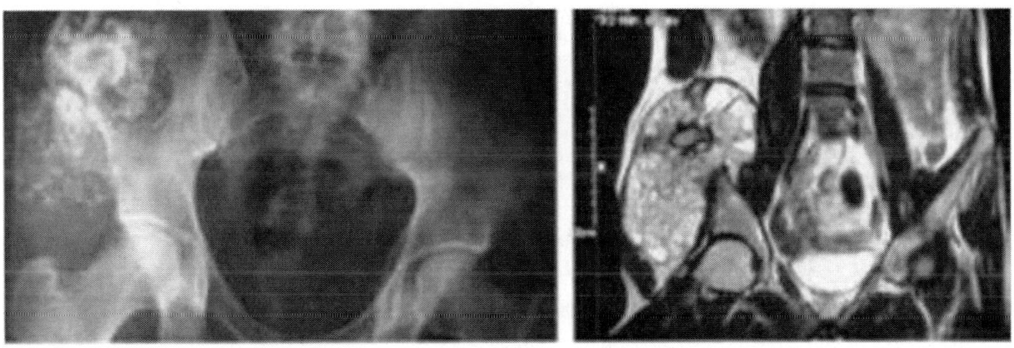

Figure 4-14. Secondary chondrosarcoma on previous pelvic exostosis. Left: A plain radiograph shows chondroid calcification. Right: MRI. Dark areas represent calcification and light areas correspond to cartilage.

EWING'S SARCOMA (EMS)

Definition

A malignant tumor originates from bone, which is made up of small round cells.

Epidemiology

- About 9% of all primary malignant tumors of the bone.
- Under 10 years is the first primary malignant bone tumor.
- It is the second primary malignant bone tumor under 30 years of age.
- It is the fourth most common primary malignant bone tumor. The third malignant non-malignant primary hematologic bone.

- M = F is reported to be slightly more common in some male studies.
- Mostly observed between 5 and 25 years old.
- About 80% are observed under the age of 20 and the rest between the ages of 20 and 30.
- The maximum age peak is 10 to 15 years old.
- It is very rare in blacks and Asians.

Site

- The most common sites of metaphyseal involvement are the long bones (often extending to the diaphysis) and the broad bones of the pelvic and girdle. The most common bone involved is the ilium, followed by the femur and fibula. The ribs are also commonly affected and their involvement can be associated with pleural effusion, and the tibia and humerus are not common bones for involvement.
- Long bone shafts, hips, and ribs are common sites of conflict.
- Metaphysis is more involved than diaphysis.
- 90% are solitary at emergence.
- All bones with red bone marrow may be involved.

Signs

- Pain is a symptom observed in all patients.
- The pain may persist for a long time before the patient sees a doctor. In one study, 50 percent of patients had symptoms for six months or more before diagnosis.
- The delay to diagnosis in a study was 34 weeks, of which 19 weeks were related to the delay in the patient's diagnostic process.
- Swelling and sometimes local heat can be observed.
- Constitutional symptoms may exist, especially when metastatic. Symptoms include fever, increased ESR and CRP, anemia, weight loss, and leukocytosis. These are late symptoms. Most patients with Ewing, like patients with osteosarcoma, do not have systemic symptoms.
- May be mistaken for osteomyelitis, especially when the tissue necrosis gives a purulent appearance to the tumor.
- Needle aspiration may be as obvious as pus, so histopathology is indicated in all suspected specimens and cultures are performed in all suspected specimens.

Imaging

- Radiography underestimate the lesion.
- A moth-eaten or permeative appearance in the diaphysis or metadiaphysis of the long bones, or in the flat bone, with a periosteal reaction, is the usual agonism of this tumor.

- Periosteal reaction in 85% is onion skin. Sometimes hair on end or sunburst or Codma'n triangle can be observed.
- A large density with an indeterminate margin is commonly observed in soft tissue, which is related to the large-tissue component of the tumor.
- Sclerotic appearance is sometimes observed with lytic or alone, which is due to reactive ossification. This condition is especially evident in metaphyseal tumors.
- Pathological fractures are observed in 10 to 15% of the cases.
- Cortex saucerization can be observed due to the soft tissue component pressure. The association of this view with the large soft tissue mass and the permeative view strongly suggests Ewing's diagnosis.
- PNET pathological fractures, metastasis, and EWS epiphyseal involvement are more common.
- Although there is no Skip metastasis in Ewing unlike osteosarcoma, all bone may be involved with the tumor.

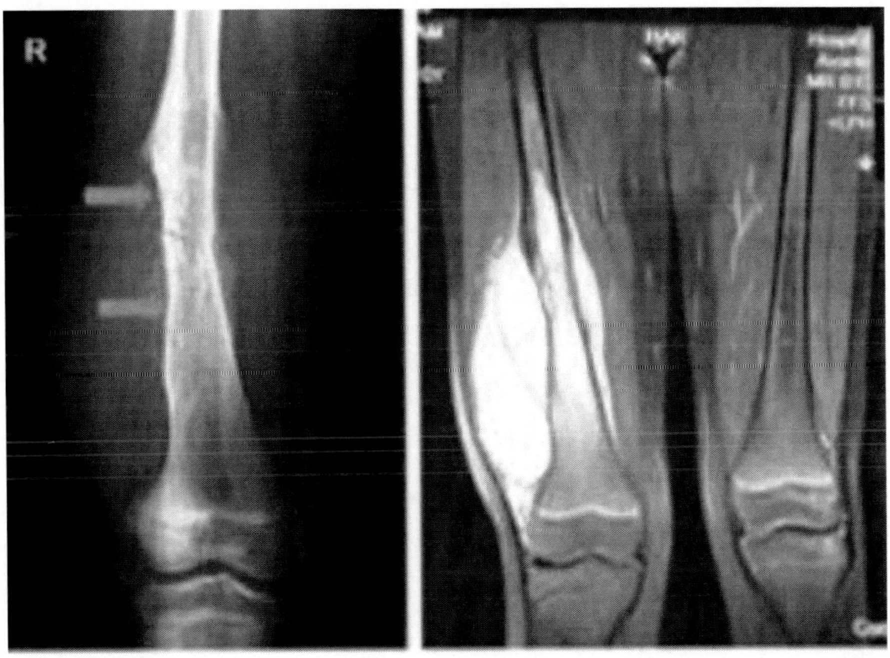

Figure 4-15. Ewing distal femoral sarcoma of the right femur. Left image: plain radiography. The arrows show the excessive pressure of the soft tissue component on the bone cortex, which has caused the cauterization of the cortex. There is a pathological fracture between the two arrows. The image on the right. MRI of T2, indicating the bulky component of soft tissue around the femur.

MRI

- The best modality for diagnosis for tumor spread to the bone marrow, soft tissue mass, skip metastasis, and response to treatment.
- Skip metastasis is more common in Osteosarcoma than EWS.
  - T1: low → intermediate
  - T2: Intermediate → high

- Lack of severe reactive edema overestimates the involvement of the medullary canal by the tumor.
- Hair on end hair loss in T2 is observed as low signal lines.

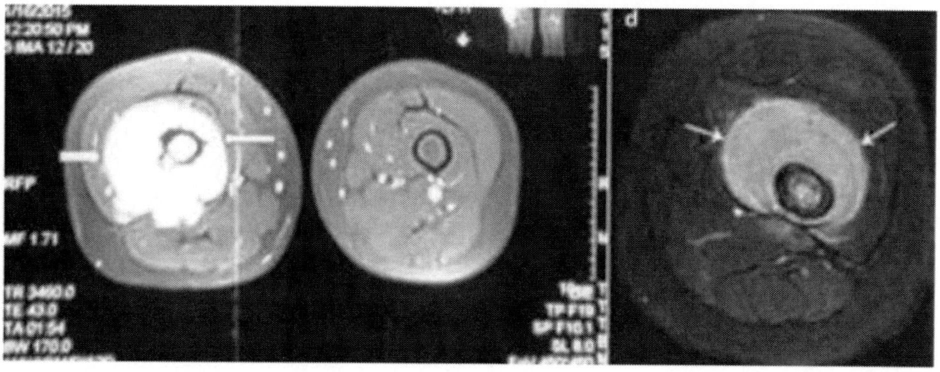

Figure 4-16. Two examples of Ewing femoral sarcoma. In both images of axial T2 MRI with fat suppressor, the arrows represent the bulky component of the tumor soft tissue, around the femoral shaft.

Bone Scan

- It has increases in absorption.
- Soft tissue mass is observed in the blood pool stage.
- Increased activity on gallium 67 scans that might show soft tissue components, can be used to assess response to treatment.
- FDG PET is highly sensitive in detecting metastasis and assessing response to treatment.

Staging

- Radiography and MRI of the primary focus.
- Chest CT + CXR.
- Bone scintigraphy.
- Bone Marrow Biopsy (BMB).
- CBC, ESR, and biochemistry.

Prognosis

- Distant metastasis is the worst prognostic factor and is only 20% if there is long-term survival.
- The size of the initial lesion is also important, but there is no definite criteria yet. Some studies have suggested a size larger than 100 cm^3 and others a diameter greater than 8 cm in the poor prognosis.
- The site of the lesion is also important, but it is difficult to differentiate it by size because proximal tumors are also larger and are both associated with poor prognosis.
- Histological grade does not have prognostic significance because all Ewings have a high grade.
- Fever, anemia, elevated LDH, WBC, ESR are associated with a poor prognosis.
- Higher age in the time of diagnosis (up to 12 to 15 years),

- Males are associated with a poor prognosis.
- More than 90% of postoperative chemotherapy necrosis, like osteosarcoma, has a good prognosis.
- The type of chromosomal displacement has no effect on prognosis.
- Recurrence in the first year after treatment like osteosarcoma, is associated with a poor prognosis.
- 5-year survival in case of local recurrence is 20% and in the case of distant metastasis is 10%.

Malignancy Potential

- In the onset 15 to 30% macrometastasis (Lung> bone) and all have micrometastasis.
- There is a 10-30% chance of secondary sarcoma in the radiotherapy field up to twenty years after radiotherapy.

Other

- Unlike other bone sarcomas, bone marrow aspiration in Ewing's sarcoma is recommended to detect systemic involvement if present. This complication occurs in 20% of patients.
- Can go beyond S.I. season.
- In very young children, acute leukemia and metastatic neuroblastoma has to be ruled out (made in the differential diagnosis).
- Over 30 years, large cell lymphoma and small cell carcinoma and myeloma has to be ruled out (they are differentiated).

Macroscopic Pathology

- It is a gray to white mass inside a modular canal with a definite margin.
- Complete rupture of the cortex is uncommon, but small cavities are more common due to tumor nests.
- The soft tissue component is often larger than the size of the lesion inside the bone. This component is often spindle-shaped and is involved around the bone.

Microscopic Pathology

- Roundcell is the head of the category of non-hematologic tumors.
- Cells do not grow densely in the sheets or nests that fill the spaces between the trabeculae.
- The cells nucleus is central and round and their cytoplasm is indistinct and insignificant.
- The most common chromosomal shift observed in more than 90% of Ewing's sarcomas is (q22; q12) (11,22)t and is diagnostic for Ewing. The most definitive diagnostic method is to show this chromosomal transmission, which can be done with PCR or fluorescent incisor hybridization.
- CD99 Coloring is prognostic for Ewing.

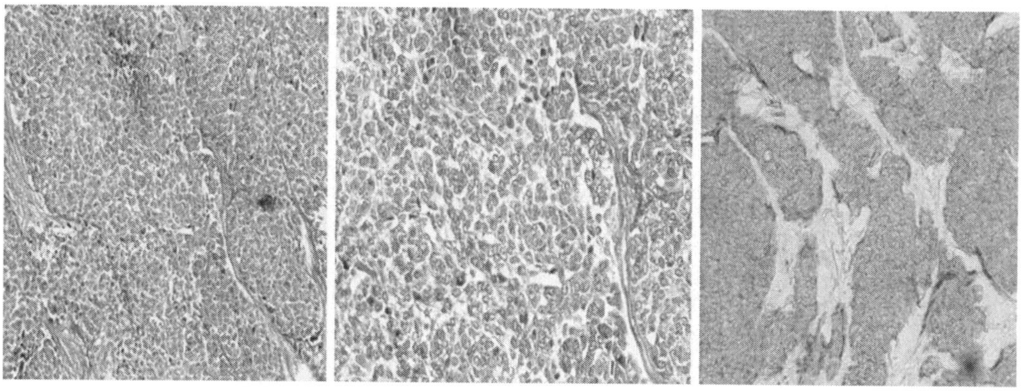

Figure 4-17. Ewing sarcoma: Cells grow in dense sheets or nests with a small central nucleus and round cytoplasm. CD99 staining (right image).

Treatment

- Extensive resection surgery with radiotherapy is combined with multidrug chemotherapy.
- With the above treatment, the 5-year life expectancy for the localized and resectable disease is 70% at diagnosis and in widespread cases is 30% at diagnosis.
- If the tumor volume is less than 100 cm^3 at the time of diagnosis, the 3-year survival of the patient is about 3 times when the tumor volume is more than 100 cm^3.
- The choice of surgery or radiotherapy for localized tumor control can vary depending on the patient.
- Surgery is preferred if extensive resection with acceptable functional impairment is possible.
- If extensive resection is impossible or is associated with an unacceptable functional defect, primary lesion radiotherapy is an acceptable alternative. As radiotherapy may be the ultimate treatment for localized tumor control, cortical defect has to be avoided when performing a biopsy to diagnose patients with suspected Ewing sarcoma and a biopsy of the tumor soft tissue component has to be sampled for biopsy.
- Radiotherapy two centimeters beyond the intraosseous extension of Ewing's sarcoma has the same effect as whole bone radiotherapy. Depending on the size of the tumor, radiotherapy is associated with ten to thirty percent of tumor recurrence. Five to thirty percent of Ewing's survivors who have received radiotherapy develop a secondary malignancy.
- Radiotherapy can be used after a marginal resection or when a large resection margin is infected.
- Like osteosarcoma, resection of pulmonary metastasis improves prognosis.
- Briefly, radiotherapy is recommended for the local control of tumor in the treatment of Ewing in the sacrum, spine, or acetabulum. In the pelvis after neoadjuvant chemotherapy, if the tumor remains large, preliminary radiotherapy is performed and then for local control of the tumor is not established, radiotherapy is selected as the final treatment for local control of the tumor. However, if the tumor volume is significantly reduced with radiotherapy, surgery is used as the final treatment for local control of the tumor.

- For the treatment of metastatic Ewing, intensification of existing chemotherapy regimens for non-metastatic Ewing or bone marrow transplantation is used. Radiotherapy is also used to control the lesion locally.

Differential Diagnosis of Ewing Sarcoma

PNET: Epiphyseal involvement, pathological Fx, and metastasis are more common.

- Osteomyelitis and eosinophilic granuloma: can be indistinguishable from radiographs of Ewing's sarcoma. They are clinically similar. Their soft tissue mass is smaller than EWS.
- Osteosarcoma: Metaphyseal, Codman's triangle and sunburst radiological view is more common.
- Lymphoma: A soft tissue mass. It can occur at the same age. They are similar in radiography.
- Metastatic neuroblastoma: Observed in children under 5 years of age.

CHORDOMA

Definition

- It is a slow-growing neoplasm that has differentiated neoplasms and is often found in the sacrococcygeal or sphenoxypital.

Origin

- It originates from the remains of embryonic notochord.
- It has physaliphorous vacuole cells and intracellular mucoid material.
- Three forms:
  - Conventional
  - Chondroid
  - Dedifferntional

Epidemiology

- It accounts for 4% of all primary malignant bone tumors.
- It is the fourth primary malignant tumor of the bone, after osteosarcoma, chondrosarcoma and Ewing's sarcoma.
- It is the second primary malignant tumor of the bone in the spine (after myeloma).
- The first primary malignant tumor is in the sacrum.
- M ÷ F = 3.
- The sacrococcygeal type is most commonly observed in the 5th to 7th decades.

- The spherocytosis type is observed in the fourth to sixth decades.
- Rarely observed in the first and second decades, in which it is typically found in the cervical vertebra.
- It is rare in blacks.

Site

- It is observed entirely in the axial skeleton.
- Sacrococcygeal is involved in more than 50% of the cases. Mostly involved below S3.
- The base of the skull is involved in 30% of the cases.
- Pythonasal spongiform encephalopathy is involved in 25% (mostly clivus) cases.
- Thoracic spine is rarely affected.
- It is centered in the body of the nut. It does not involve posterior and disc elements and is usually extradural.

Clinical Signs

- It varies depending on the site and extent of the tumor.
- There have been nonspecific symptoms for months to years.
- Sphenococcal: Headache, cranial nerve pulsation, an endocrine disorder due to pressure on the pituitary gland, mimicking the symptoms of Cp angle tumor, bleeding and nasal obstruction can be observed.
- Spine: Compresses the cord or nerve.
- Sacrococcygeal: Back pain is the most common complaint.
- Sciatica, paresthesia, anorectal or bladder dysfunction can be observed.
- On rectal examination, the mass is commonly palpable.

Imaging

- As a single lytic lesion, it is dilated and severely destructive of the axial skeleton.
- The site of the tumor in the coronal view is in the midline.
- The tumor is better observed on the lateral radiograph than on the ap view, because it is difficult to see the tumor in the view of the intestinal gas.
- A large soft tissue mass is observed along with the bone marrow.
- It may have a sclerotic rim, intracranial calcification, and pathological fractures.
- The environment of the lesion is irregular with a scalloping mode.
- It can affect several vertebral segments but does not involve the discs.
- It can be paramedian. It can be sclerotic.
- Intracellular calcification is observed in more than 50% of the cases.
- CT is the best modality to show:
    - Bony margins

- ▪ Bone fragmentation (intra-tumor calcification)

MRI

- It is best to show the full extent of the lesion and its relationship to other anatomical structures.
- A soft tissue mass is observed.
- It has lobulated border.
- It moves the bladder and intestines but does not invade them.
- T1: Low → intermediate
- T2: High heterogeneous
- Heterogenous Gadolinium enhancement
- Very high signal T2: This is only the case when it is myxoid.

BS

- Accumulation of radioisotope fluid in the bladder may prevent the tumor from being observed on a nuclear scan.
- Decreased absorption in the center.
- Increases absorption in the environment.

Malignancy Tendency

- Slow growth, local aggressive, recurrent recurrence.
- Long-term prognosis is bad.

Macroscopic Pathology

- It is a gray-gray multi-lobcd soft mass.
- Commonly have a myxoid or gelatinous appearance.
- A thin layer of periosteum covers the area of the dilated bone.
- The bony inner part of the tumor has an indeterminate margin.

Microscopic Pathology

- It is observed as cell lobes separated by fibrous bands.
- Cells have an abundant vacuolated cytoplasm and are formed as nests or cords inside the myxoid stroma.
- The nucleus of the cells is round or oval.
- Nucleus Pleomorphism is obvious.
- The undifferentiated type includes areas with high-grade sarcoma (mostly MFH) and is more aggressive.

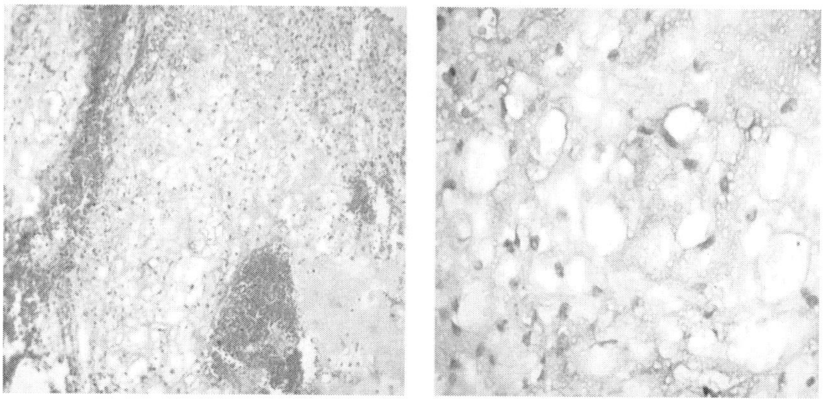

Figure 4-18. Chordoma: Cells have an abundant vacuolated cytoplasm and are formed as nests or cords inside the myxoid stroma.

Treatment

- Extensive resection is the treatment of choice even if it leads to a neurological defect.
- Some believe that complete resection of the tumor is the treatment of choice if possible.
- Non-resectable tumors are treated with blockage and radiotherapy.
- In case of infection of the operating environment with the tumor, treatment is optional.
- Non-resectable tumors are treated with blockage and radiotherapy.
- If the operating environment becomes infected with a tumor, radiotherapy is prescribed.
- Imatinib is used for a wide range of diseases.
- Distant metastasis is observed late. Lungs, bones, lymph nodes, brain, kidneys, liver, eyelids and skin are common sites of metastasis. 10% of patients find in distant.
- The average survival of patients is generally 4 years.
- If the roots of S2 and S3 on both sides are preserved, urinary and fecal control will remain, and resecting S2 on both sides will result in complete loss of urinary and fecal control.
- Chemotherapy has no proven effect on treatment.

Other

- Rarely observed as soft tissue mass without bone involvement.
- Good prognosis:
  - Male gender
  - Young age of the patient
  - Distal lesion in the sacrococcygeal

DD

- Chondrosarcoma: Shows the arcs & rings of the chondroid calcification.
- Metastasis: Soft tissue mass is less common in metastasis.
- Plasmacytoma: Rarely positive on bone scan.
- Osteomyelitis, lymphoma: Clinical information helps to differentiate.
- GCT sarcoma is more proximal to chordoma.

ADAMANTINOMA

Definition

- A rare malignant neoplasm of the lower extremity with a biphasic histological appearance in the tibia and rarely fibula.
- Histologically, it is similar to maxillary adamantinoma, which is a much more common tumor.

Epidemiology

- It is rare. Less than 1% of primary bone tumors.
- Average age 35-25 years. Rarely observed under 20 years.
- M> F.

Site

- 90% in tibia. It is almost always located in the anterior cortex.
- Up to 50% of fibula lesions occur simultaneously.
- Diaphysis is the most common site (70%) and then metadiaphysis is the next most common.

About 10-20% of the cases are observed in other bones of the body except the tibia and fibula depending on various reports.

Clinical Signs

- The most common symptoms are pain and deformity over months – years.
- Thunder masses, fixed and firm may exist.
- Anterior cortical involvement and moderate to severe curvature are typically observed in the tibia.
- There is no curvature in the fibula, but bone dilatation is typical.

Imaging

- 70% of tumors are located in the tibial shaft.
- 30% are observed at both ends of the tibia.
- The margin is distinct, lytic, and sclerotic, mixed longitudinally parallel to the longitudinal axis of the bone diaphysis, centered in the anterior tibial cortex and has a lobular margin. Lucent lesions have a definite margin.
- 80% is larger than 5 cm.

- Mostly extends into the medulla of the canal.
- Destruction of cortex with the serrated view is specific.
- Multifocal satellite lesions within the bone are histologically along the main lesion but are radiologically separate from the main lesion.
- Growth is slow.

MRI

- Soft tissue proliferation occurs in 90% of the cases.
- Expansion to medullary canal may exist.
- T1: Low → intermediate.
- T2: High homogeneous/heterogeneous.

BS

- Increased absorption.

The potential for malignancy

- Local aggressive.
- 10-year life span is 10 to 65%.

Macroscopic Pathology

- It is as a soft and fleshy mass.
- It can be multifocal or involve a large segment of the medullary canal.
- Gradual conversion from fleshy, soft to firm, and fibrous can be observed.
- Complete destruction of the cortex and invasion of the surrounding soft tissue can be observed.

Microscopic Pathology

- Classical adamantinoma involves large nests or masses of epithelial tumor cells.
- Contains epithelial cells in the stroma of fibrosis or fibro-osseous.
- Around the nests, there are layers of cubic cells that are more or less perpendicular to the mass of internal epithelial cells.

Treatment

- Extensive resection and extensive reconstruction and rehabilitation of standard organs is the standard treatment.
- Local recurrence (25%) and pulmonary metastasis (30%) may occur years later, so long-term clinical and radiological follow-up is required.
- The treatment for local recurrence is amputation.
- The ten-year life expectancy of these patients after successful surgery with a wide margin is 80 to 90%.

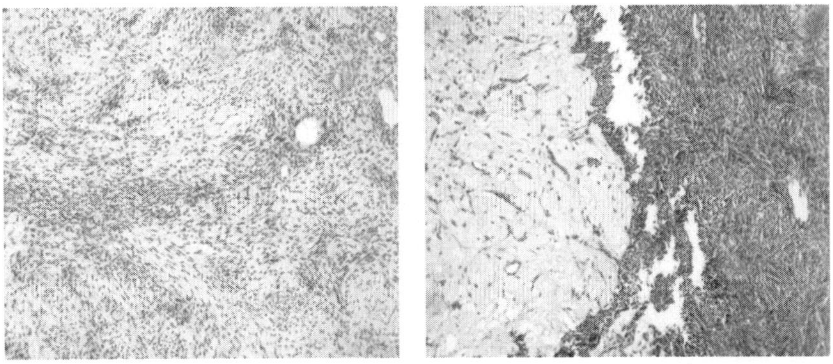

Figure 4-19. Adamantinoma: Biphasic tumor, Classical adamantinoma involves large nests or masses of epithelial tumor cells. Contains epithelial cells in the stroma of fibrosis or fibro-osseous.

Other

- Adamantinoma has to be considered for any cortical lesion of the anterior tibial cortex, even if it is small, non-invasive with slow growth.
- It is important to have a biopsy from the center of the tumor because there is more epithelium in the center. The presence of epithelium is necessary for diagnosis.
- Paraneoplastic hyperemia has been observed in adamantinoma.
- Extensive destruction of the cortex is often present.
- 23% present with pathological Fx as the first manifestation.
- In various studies with 5 to 10 years follow-up, local recurrence was between 20 to 30% and metastasis was 12 to 22%.
- The difference between osteofibrous dysplasia adamantinoma and adamantinoma:
  - The incidence of osteofibrous dysplasia-like adamantinoma is (the first two decades of life).
  - osteofibrous dysplasia-like adamantinoma is intra-cortical
  - There is a small site of epithelial cells in the pathology of osteofibrous dysplasia-like adamantinoma.
- Histological signs in favor of diagnosing adamantinoma:
  - Keratin cyst
  - Desmosome
  - Differential Diagnosis
- Osteofibrosis dysplasia: Younger and older patients have a definite margin, are less invasive unless they are small.
- FD (fibrous dysplasia): is more central in the medullary canal. It has a ground glass view.
- NOF: In younger patients, the bulk of the tumor rests in the medullary canal.
- Osteomyelitis: Seek sequestrum and periosteal reaction.
- For further reading:
  - Article June 2010 AAOS vol 18 No 6

Fibrous Tumors

Fibrosarcoma

Definition

- Malignant neoplasms are spindle-shaped cells that differentiate into myofibroblasts.

Epidemiology

- Uncommon. 5% of all malignant primary bone tumors. It is observed from the second decade to the seventh decade. The maximum prevalence is in the fifth decade of life.
- M = F

Source

25% is secondary to:

- Radiotherapy
- Paget's disease
- Bone infarction
- Chronic osteomyelitis

Site

- Long bone metaphysis is the most common site of tumor involvement.
- 50% of the cases are found in the distal femur or proximal tibia.
- It can also spread to the epiphysis.

Clinical Signs

- Pain is the most common initial finding.
- Local swelling and tenderness may exist.
- Occurs in 19% with pathological fractures.

X-Ray

- It is completely lytic with an indistinct margin and a permeative or moth-eaten appearance.
- No sclerosing margin.
- Cortex destruction and soft tissue spread are often observed.

- Periost ossification and Cadman triangle may be observed.
- Bony sequestrum is present.
- In children, the open phase prevents the tumor from entering the epiphysis but after the tumor closes, the tumor can spread to the epiphysis.

MRI

- T1: Low → intermediate.
- T2: Intermediate → high.
- Increased absorption with Gadolinium is heterogeneous.
- Increases peripheral absorption in bone scans.

Malignancy Potential

- Tends to local recurrence and metastasis.
- favorable radiological view:
  - Eccentric
  - Geographical view
  - Involve less than half of the bone environment.
- Poor prognosis:
  - Age over 40 years.
  - Axial skeleton
  - high-grade tumor
- Lung metastasis are particularly common and will occur in 45% of the cases.
- 10-year survival:
  - Low grade 83%.
  - High grade 34%.

Macroscopic Pathology

- Tan-gray color with foci of bleeding and necrosis.
- It has a meaty consistency.

Microscopic Pathology

- Parallel clusters of uniform spindle-shaped cells in the shape of herringbone are characteristic of this tumor.

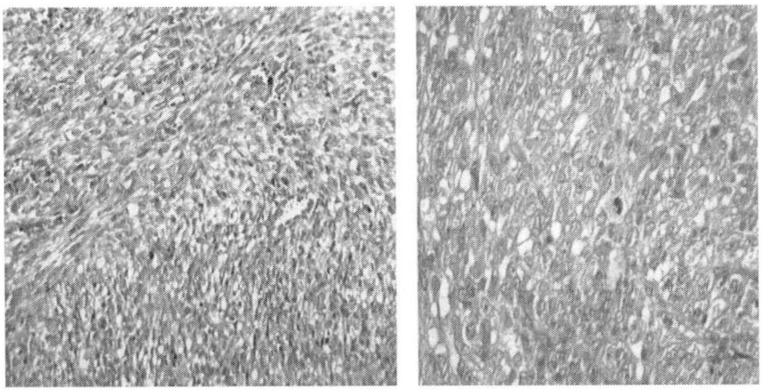

Figure 4-20. Fibrosarcoma bundles of tumor cells arranged in the shape of a herringbone.

Treatment

- For low grade wide excision or Amputation.
- For high grade, the treatment is similar to MFH treatment.

Other

- The following has to be considered in any aggression lesion with sequestrum (small cortical or trabecular bone fragments within the aggression lytic lesion):
  - Osteomyelitis
  - Fibrosarcoma
  - MFH
  - Lymphoma
  - LCH
- Calcification in the margin or inside of fibrosarcoma indicates fibrosarcoma arising from a bone infarct.

DD

- MFH: Both may have sequestra.
- Chondrosarcoma: Has a chondroid matrix.
- GCT: It is an epiphysis and extends to the subchondral bone.
- DF: It is more geographical in radiology.
- EWS: Has a larger soft tissue mass. It is more likely to contain a sclerotic component inside the bone and new periosteal ossification. Cortical saucerization may occur.
- LCH: More likely to have new multi-layered periosteal ossification.

MFH

Another name: Undifferentiated high grade pleomorphic sarcoma

Epidemiology

- It is Rare and consists of 2% of primary bone malignancies.
- Observed from the second to the seventh decade.
- Higher incidence in people over 50 years of age.
- M> F (slightly).

Source

- It is a malignant tumor of fibeocyctic cells.
- Spiral pattern of fibroblasts, histiocytes, and pleomorphic cells.
- Secondary includes 28% of the cases.

- Paget
- Bone infarct
- Irritation
- Chondrosarcoma
- Parosteal osteosarcoma.
- Low-grade osteosarcoma.
- Chronic osteomyelitis
- GCT
- Diaphyseal medullary stenosis: The diaphyseal medullary canal is narrow and the cortex is thick. 30% of patients with this autosomal dominant syndrome will develop MFH.

Site

- 90% in metaphysis of long bones, which commonly extend to the epiphysis and they are central.
- It is mostly around the knee.
- Femur (45% - 30) ← Tibia ← Homer ← Iliak.
- Those originating in the diaphysis are eccentric.

Clinical Signs

- Pain with less prevalence of swelling (average 7-9 months).
- In 20% of the cases, it occurs with pathological fractures.

Imaging

- It is mostly metaphyseal. Diaphysis involvement is less common.
- It has a completely lytic appearance with an indeterminate margin.
- Usually a geographical view is visible. A permeative view can also be observed.
- In the early stages, there is destruction of the cortex and soft tissue expansion.
- No periosteal reaction except in cases of fractures.
- Mineralization may be observed only at the periphery of the soft tissue component.
- Intracellular calcification is rare.

MRI

- T1: Low → intermediate.
- T2: Fat suppressed and T2: Heterogenous intermediate-high.
- Increased absorption of Gadolinium is heterogeneous and more intense in the environment.

BS

- Increased absorption in the intraosseous part of the lesion for unknown reasons.
- Ga67 is more sensitive than Tc99 for primary lesions and metastasis.

Malignant potential

- High probability.
- The secondary type is more aggressive than the primary type.

Macroscopic Pathology

- Tan-gray with fleshy and yellow areas.
- Focal points of bleeding and necrosis are common.
- Tumor consistency varies from soft to fibrous and hard.

Microscopic Pathology

- Spindle cells with a tornado pattern are the main features of this tumor.
- It has areas of pleomorphic cells.
- The amount of collagen in the tumor matrix varies.

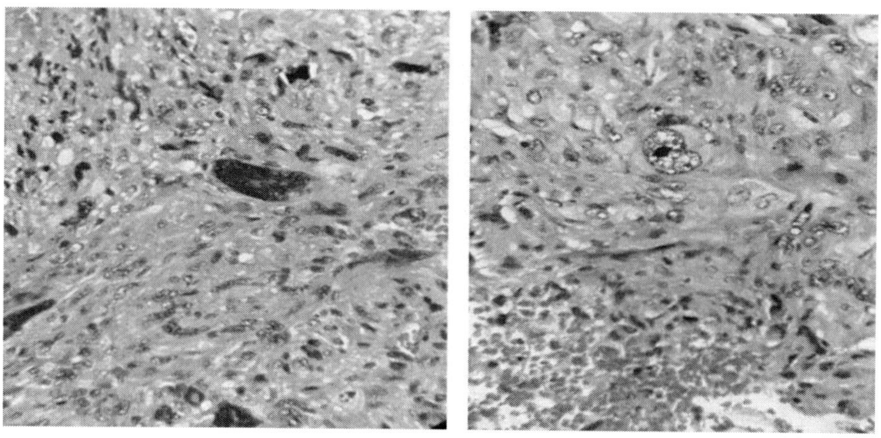

Figure 4-21. MFH: Pleomorphic spindle cells are characteristic of this tumor.

Treatment

- Wide excision along with chemotherapy, radiotherapy is the basis of treatment.
- 5-year survival with the above method is 67%.
- Half of the patients will have lung metastasis.
- Localized lymph node metastasis is observed in 4%.
- 10-year lifespan is 36% in the secondary type and 46% in the primary type.
- The percentage of necrosis is of prognostic importance.

Other

- The secondary type to bone infarct begins its destruction from the environment.
- Joint invasion is observed in 30% of MRIs.

DD

It is similar to fibrosarcoma.

Epithelioid hemangioma and endothelium.

Definition

- It is a well-differentiated endothelial vascular neoplasm whose endothelial cells have an epithelial appearance and tend to be focal.

Epidemiology

- It is very rare.
- Its peak age is in the second and third decade.
- It is obviously more common in males than in females.

Common Site

- Any bone can be affected, but the bones of the lower extremities, including the foot bones, are more affected.
- The tibia is the most common bone involved.
- Most patients initially have multiple bone conflicts, which tend to involve the bones of one area of the body or one limb.
- Simultaneous involvement of silent bones such as the tibia and fibula is common.
- Unlike hemangiomas, the spine is not involved.

Imaging

- It is characterized as a completely lytic lesion with different amounts of sclerosis at its periphery.
- The margins of the lesion are clear.
- Cortical erosion or complete rupture may be observed.
- In rare cases, a willow or permeative appearance may be observed.
- It does not have periosteal ossification and soft tissue invasion is rare.
- The presence of several lytic foci and the tendency to trap the bones of one limb is the key to diagnosis.
- In rare cases, it can be made of plastic.

Macroscopic Pathology

- The extent of the lesion is known from healthy tissue but is irregular in the environment and is associated with scalloping.
- The contents of the tumor are red and sometimes gelatinous in the form of soft bleeding tissue.

Microscopic Pathology

- It is made up of rigid nests made up of cords of epithelial cells that sometimes form narrow vascular spaces.

- Epithelioid cells may be scattered throughout the area.
- The supporting connective tissue (stroma) of the tumor is myxoid or cartilaginous.
- They are round or polygonal cells.
- Mitotic activity is low.
- The cytoplasm is eosinophilic and contains vacuoles.
- The nuclei are round and the nuclei are clear.

Treatment

- There is no agreement on a definitive treatment strategy for this tumor.
- Some cases have been treated with en block resection and some with curettage.
- Used in cases of multifocal radiotherapy.
- In general, due to gradual progression, this tumor can be treated with limited surgery along with radiofrequency ablation and radiotherapy.
- Intraosseous angiosarcoma

Definition

- Moderate to high-grade malignant tumors include atypical endothelial cells that have an angiogenic appearance. Neoplastic blood vessels are covered with a layer of malignant endothelial cells.

Other Names

- Hemangioendothelioma, hemangiosarcoma, vascular sarcoma, and epithelioid angiosarcoma.

Epidemiology

- Very rare.
- M = F.
- It is observed in equal proportions from the second to the eighth decade.

Site

- 60% is found in long bones. It is more common in the lower extremities and Then it is common in Spine is common.
- Typically an area of bone is involved, but multifocal cases have also been reported.
- One-third of the cases are multifocal, especially in the lower extremities.

Clinical Signs

- Local pain and swelling.
- Sometimes pathological fracture.

Imaging

- Destructive lytic with irregular margins is observed.
- Degradation of the cortex and spread into the soft tissue is observed in high-grade lesions.
- With radiography, a benign tumor cannot be distinguished from a malignant one.
- Lytic lesions (one or more) near the end of the bone, with an indistinct margin and varying in size.
- High-grade lesions destroy the cortex and soft tissue mass.
- Lesions with a lower grade have a sclerotic rim.
- Simultaneous involvement of several bones in one limb or in an anatomical area with a honeycomb appearance is in favor of the vascular nature of the lesion.
- Skeletal survey: Recommended due to the possibility of being multifocal and the risk of pathological fractures.
- In angiography, a mass with high absorption and a certain margin is observed along with the presence of shunts and veins that drain the contrast material quickly.
- CT: Nonspecific.
- In MRI: Unlike hemangiomas, the component has no fat. Infiltrative lesion is nonspecific.
- On MRI: Serpentine vessels are often found in the lesion environment and look like all vessels as follows:
  - High-velocity blood vessels are dark in both T2 & T1 views.
  - Veins with low blood flow velocity are bright in T2 view
- Bone scan: Increases absorption.

Microscopic Pathology

- Irregular vascular cyst-like spaces covered with atypical endothelial cells.
- Epithelial endothelial cells are observed in the form of nests, cords, or blades.
- It is composed of atypical endothelial cells.
- Irregular anastomotic vessels lined with obese endothelial cells are observed.
- Nuclear atypia is evident in high-grade tumors.
- Endothelial cells often germinate inside the lumen of the vessel.
- The higher the grade of the tumor, the more invisible the angiogenesis and the fewer endothelial markers.
- Epithelial markers are less common in low-grade tumors.

Differential Diagnosis

- Hemangioma: have lower infiltrative border and show fat overgrowth.
- Kaposi's sarcoma, metastasis, myeloma: no visible vessels on MRI.
- Bacillary angiomatosis: observed in AIDS, is associated with common skin lesions, has systemic symptoms, and is associated with a periosteal reaction.
- Cystic angiomatosis: Similar to angiosarcoma but symptoms of visceral involvement are common. Usually occurs in the spine.

Treatment

- Radical surgery in the form of excision or amputation is recommended.
- Radiotherapy and chemotherapy have been used, although there is no significant evidence to support their effectiveness.

Other

- Can be observed at the site of previous radiotherapy, bone infarction, or fibrous dysplasia.
- Kasabach-Merrit syndrome is associated with hemangioma, hemangioendothelioma, or angiosarcoma with thrombocytopenia and purpura with intravascular coagulation, bleeding diathesis, and arthropathy due to recurrent hemarthrosis.
- Aspiration or needle biopsy of vascular lesions is often undiagnosed and carries a risk of bleeding.
- Secondary angiosarcoma has been observed in the following cases:
  - Bone infract.
  - Fibrous dysplasia.
  - Exposure to radioactive radiation.

PRIMARY BONE LYMPHOMA

Synonyms

Reticulum cell sarcoma.

Epidemiology

- It can be observed at any age, but is more common in the sixth and seventh decades.
- Slightly more common in men.
- Most cases are primary non-Hodgkin's lymphoma (diffuse large B cell type). Between 70 and 83%.

Types

- The primary NHL has no distant lymph nodes or soft tissue involvement and, according to some authors, has no lymph nodes or extracellular involvement for up to 6 months. Up to 6 months after diagnosis, only bone marrow lymphoma is observed.
- Secondary NHL: it is NHL metastasis, seen in 20-10% of children with lymphoma.
- Primary bone Hodgkin's is extremely rare.
- Secondary Hodgkin's disease can be observed in advanced Hodgkin's disease.

Site

- The femur is the most common site of involvement. Then the pelvis, spine, and ribs are the next common sites.
- Humerus and cranium are the next most common sites.
- In 15% of the cases, it is observed as multifocal lesions.
- In long bones, it is usually diaphyseal and near the metaphysis.

Clinical Signs

- Pain is the most common complaint.
- May be asymptomatic.
- Local tenderness, redness and swelling may also be observed.
- Unlike primary generalized lymphoma and Ewing's sarcoma, fever is rare in the early NHL.
- Some patients may have symptoms from several years before visiting by medicine.
- Unlike multiple myeloma, patients with lymphoma appear completely healthy in other ways.
- Pathological fracture may be the primary symptom.
- Pathological fractures are observed in 25% of the cases.

Imaging

Early NHL

- The lytic lesion is usually observed with a permeative or permeative appearance near the end of a long bone, with a large size and an indistinct margin.
- It is usually lytic. Rarely, it may also be plastic.
- Usually a large part of the bone and sometimes the whole of it is involved.
- Pathological fractures and soft tissue spread are common.
- Onion skin prickly reaction is common but not as common as Ewing.
- Radiography may be normal. Lymphoma is a differential diagnosis of bone pain with normal radiography and abnormal bone scan or MRI.
- Sequestrum, is observed in 16% of the cases.
- It Can cross the joint and go to the opposite side. Metastasis of thyroid carcinoma also has this feature. But in general, this feature is rare in tumors.

NHL Secondary

- Multiple (rarely single) lytic lesions with an indistinct moth-eaten margin are observed.
- It has soft tissue spreading.

Hodgkin

- 10 - 25% have radiographic findings.
- The spine, pelvis, ribs, sternum, and femur are involved.
- Ivovy vertebra is seen due to diffuse sclerosis. Sclerosis is more common in Hodgkin than non-Hodgkin
- Sclerosis, lytic, mixed lesions can be observed.
- Sclerosis is more common in secondary Hodgkin than in the secondary NHL.
- Burkitt's lymphoma specifically affects the facial bones.

Skeletal Complications Treatment

- Osteonecrosis: observed 1 to 3 years after starting chemotherapy.
- Methotrexate osteoarthropathy: has pain, osteopenia, growth recovery lines.

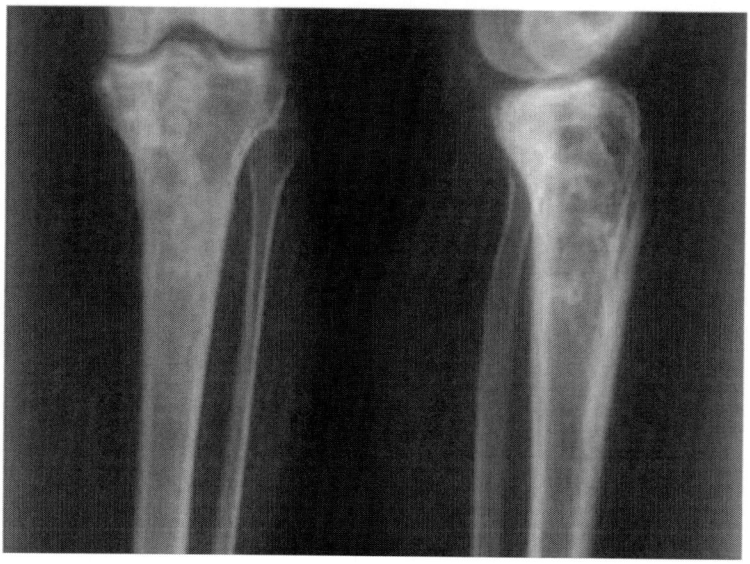

Figure 4-22. Non-Hodgkin's lymphoma in the tibia of a 28-year-old man. Notice the willow view near the end of the bone along with the blast view.

MRI

- The most accurate study for finding the bone marrow and soft tissue spreading.
- T1: Iso-intense to muscle.
- T2: Hyper-intense to muscle.
- Reactive edema around the tumor.
- Tumor spread into soft tissue (soft tissue component) could be oozing form or spreading form. The destruction of the cortex is negligible. This condition also occurs in round cell tumors. This is due to the spread of tumor cells within the Haversian Canals, which, due to their small size, do not require obvious bone destruction to enter the surrounding soft tissue.
- A small set of radiographic findings with obvious involvement of the bone marrow and surrounding soft tissue is helpful in diagnosing lymphoma.

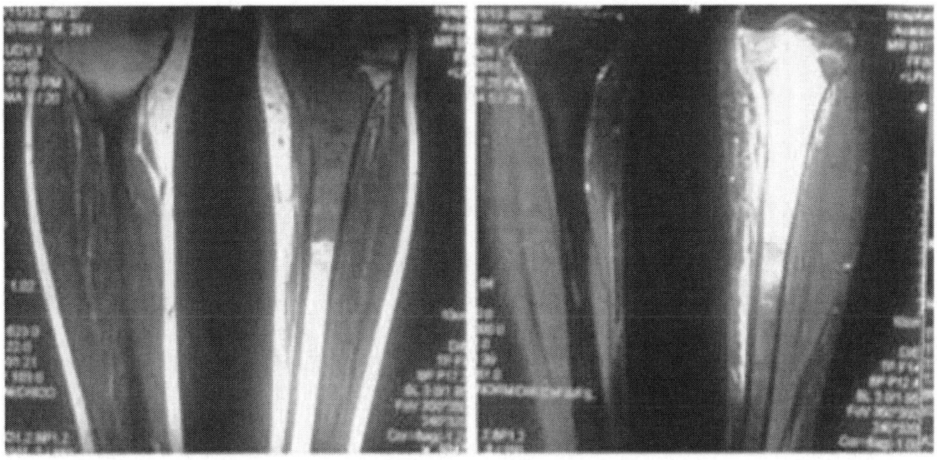

Figure 4-23. Left and right T1 and T2 MRI with fat suppressor from non-Hodgkin's lymphoma in the 28-year-old male tibia, respectively.

BS

- It is usually positive.

Staging

- Blood cell counts and biochemical tests.
- Bone scan.
- CT scan of the chest, abdomen and pelvis.
- Bone marrow aspiration.

Macroscopic Pathology

- The diffuse type with large cell, which is the most common type, is observed as a tan or white-gray flesh lesion.
- Areas of necrosis, bleeding, and cystic degeneration may exist.
- Reactive sclerosis can cover a wide area.

Microscopic Pathology

- Round cells with a diffuse growth pattern are the most common.
- Compressed tumor cells take on the appearance of a spindle cell.
- In lymphoma, specific stains are positive for CD20 & CD45, but in multiple myeloma they are negative.
- In lymphoma, reticulin staining is positive and PAS is negative. This is the opposite of Ewing.

Treatment

- The primary treatment for bone marrow lymphoma is chemotherapy.
- Local treatment is usually with radiotherapy.
- Surgery is required for fractures treatment or as a prophylaxis treatment.

- The five-year survival of primary bone lymphoma is 55%, and the systemic type is 25%.
- Age and stage of the disease are the most important prognostic factors. Patients younger than 30 years have a much better prognosis than patients older than 60 years.

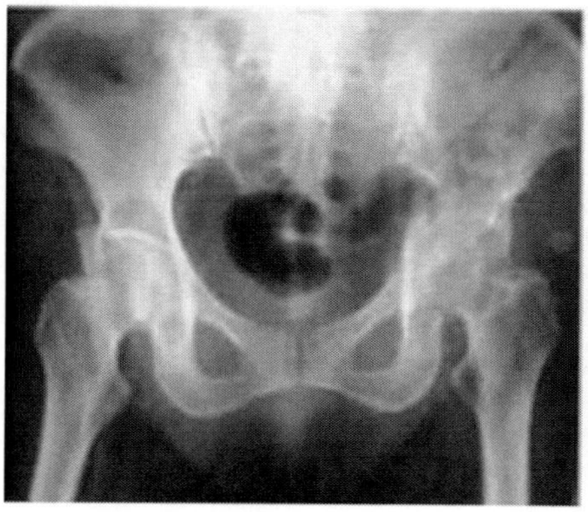
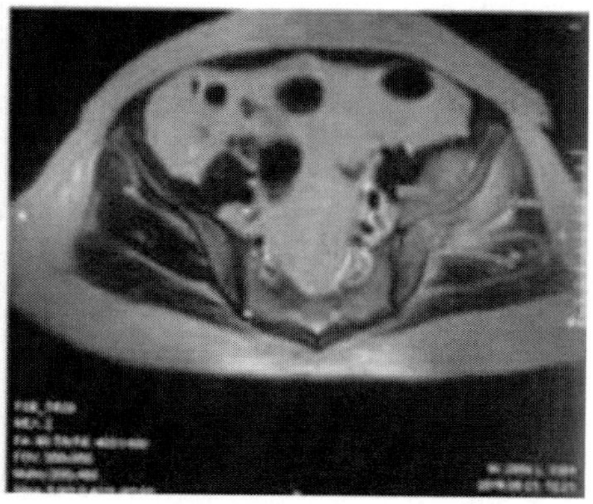

Figure 4-24. Lymphoma in the left ilium. Right: T2 view. The arrows represent the large soft tissue component of the tumor.

Other

- Primary, is always considered as stage 1 because it is limited to bone.
- Secondary, is considered stage 4 because the lesion is due to another disease elsewhere.

Differential Diagnosis

- Ewing's sarcoma, osteomyelitis, and eosinophilic granuloma: difficult to distinguish from lymphoma. In imaging, they may be similar.
- Metastasis, plasmacytoma: Moth eaten and periosteal reaction are less common.
- Paget's disease (Ivory vertebra): The vertebrae are enlarged, the cortex and trabeculae are thickened.

LEUKEMIA

Epidemiology

- All children, adolescents
- AML Adolescents, Youth
- Adult CLL, over 25 years
- Hairy cell leukemia in middle-aged men
- In all groups, men> women are affected

Clinical Signs

- Fever, bleeding, fatigue, lymphadenopathy, hepatosplenomegaly, susceptibility to infection.

Imaging

- Disseminated osteopenia. Permeative or permeative focal lytic lesions with new periosteal ossification due to subperiosteal leukemic cells. Diffuse infiltration in the bones is observed due to bone marrow involvement, which does not look like primary bone lesions.
- In children, it is observed as metaphyseal lucent bands (broad with indeterminate margin due to infiltration) or (thin and with definite margin due to osteoporosis).
- Bone infarcts and pathological fractures are also observed.

Imaging (AML, CML, CLL)

- Disseminated osteopenia.
- Focal lytic lesions.
- Chloroma, a mass of myelogenous cells that causes a lytic lesion or soft tissue mass (AML> CML).

MRI

- T1: Low → intermediate
- T2: high → .Intermediate
- Some contrast enhancement with gadolinium.
- In children, MRI evaluation can be problematic due to the hematopoietic bone marrow and increased natural vertebral absorption in children younger than 7 years of age.
- Chloroma: It has a different appearance. The margin can be clear or indistinct. The general appearance of MRI is similar to leukemia itself, but the contrast enhancement is severe.

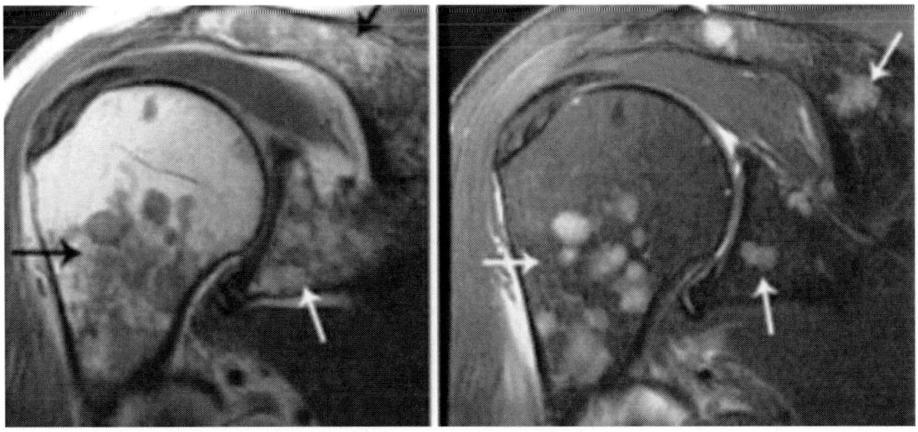

Figure 4-25. Leukemic infiltration. Left: T1 and right T2 with fat suppressor.

Treatment

- Chemotherapy for all types.
- Bone marrow transplantation for CML & AML.

Differential Diagnoses of Radiolucent Metaphysical Bands on Radiography

- Normal
- Leukemia
- Metastatic neuroblastoma
- Metabolic: Ricketts, Scurvy
- Congenital syphilis

MYELOMA

Definition

Monoclonal proliferation of neoplastic plasma cells that involve the bone marrow and rarely the extra-skeletal region.

Other Names

- Plasma cell myeloma
- Solitary plasmacytoma
- Sclerotic myeloma

Epidemiology

- The most common malignant primary bone tumor.
- It is the most common malignancy observed with skeletal lesions.
- The second one is hematopoietic malignancy.
- Mostly observed between the ages of 65 and 74.
- Less than 1% of the cases are observed in people younger than 40 years.
- It is more common in blacks.
- M = F.

Source

- Neoplastic proliferation of monoclonal plasmacells originating in the bone marrow can spread to other organs.
- Myeloma cells produce bone by stimulating the production of osteoclast stimulating factor.
- Monoclonal MGUS is always observed after gammotopathy of undetermined significance.

Site

- The most common site of axial skeletal involvement is the skull.
- Proximal limbs are the next most common.
- Only 10% is seen Distal to knee and elbow.
- It is common in areas where hematopoietic bone marrow is present in adults.

Clinical Signs

- It usually occurs as multifocal bone lytic lesions, plasma cell proliferation, and monoclonal gammopathy.
- Patients with multifocal bone pain typically have a history of recurrent infections, mostly in weight-bearing areas and spina bifida, anemia, hypercalcemia, renal failure, proteinuria, and recurrent infections.
- Weakness, fatigue, fever, weight loss, bleeding, and thrombocytopenia, neurological symptoms due to compression fracture or expansion into the soft tissue of plasma cells are other symptoms of this disease.
- Peripheral neuropathy is especially observed in osteosclerotic myeloma.
- Due to the aggressive nature of this tumor, symptoms usually appear shortly after the patient is referred.
- Hyperviscosity and symptoms of amyloidosis can also be observed.
- Increased M, Alp monoclonal component in serum or urine in 99% of individuals, monoclonal light chain in 25% (Bance Jones protein).

Recommended Tests

- Complete blood count
- Serum creatinine
- Serum calcium
- Electrophoresis of serum proteins by immunofixation
- Examination of light chain in serum
- Urine protein analysis

Imaging

- In 80% of multiple myeloma, marked changes are observed on the radiograph.
- Punched out lesions are the first and most obvious radiographic findings. Their diameter may reach a maximum of 5 cm.
- May cause endosteal scalloping, similar to bone murmur.
- Small bones, such as the ribs, may dilate and take on the appearance of a balloon.
- Has no sclerotic rim or periosteal ossification.

- In myeloma, bone scans are often negative.
- Compression fracture of the vertebrae or even the vertebrae may be the reason for the patient's visit.
- At the diagnosis, 25% to 12% have generalized osteopenia, which may be quite obvious. These individuals have no specific lytic lesions.
- In less than 3% of the cases, the radiographic appearance is completely sclerotic, observed with POEMS syndrome.
- Plasmacytoma consists of a soft tissue mass or dilated and bubble-shaped lytic lesion.

Skeletal surgery in multiple myeloma includes the following:

- Humerus
- Femurs
- Skull
- Pelvis
- Ribs
- Spine

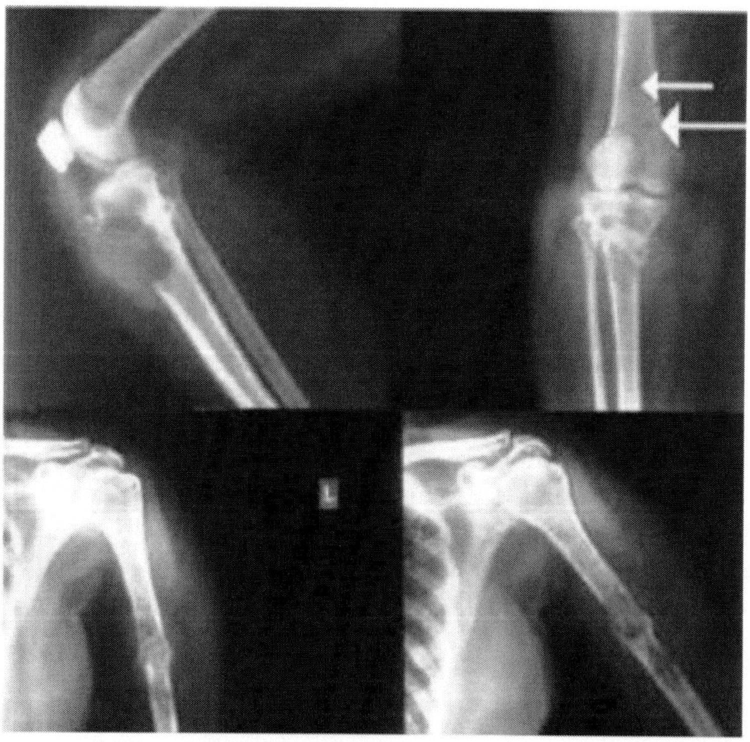

Figure 4-26. Multiple Myeloma. Lytic lesions with indeterminate margins in the proximal tibia of the humerus diaphysis. Arrows indicate punched out lesions in the distal femur.

Diagnostic Workup

- Skeletal surgery (not nuclear scan).
- B.M.B/B.M.A Bone marrow aspiration/biopsy.

- MRI: In people who have bone pain and a negative radiograph, or an initial diagnosis of a single bone plasmacytoma.
- PET is not routinely recommended.

MRI

- It is more sensitive than radiography, CT and nuclear scan, but less sensitive than radiography in the ribs. It may be normal or the focal lesions may look metastatic.
- The response to treatment is determined by:
  - Nonenhancement with or without radiographic lesion
  - In T2 the increase of the signal becomes the decrease of the signal.

Macroscopic Pathology

- It is composed of soft gray-gray texture.
- Diffuse involvement of the bone marrow is observed in the form of multiple nodules at autopsy.

Microscopic Pathology

- At least one subset of cells resembles normal plasmas.
- Tumor cells form lumps or clumps in the bone marrow.
- The cells are round or oval with an eccentric nucleus.
- If multiple myeloma is suspected, a smear has to always be obtained, as the nature of the infiltration of round-infiltrated plasma cells is better determined in cytology than histology.

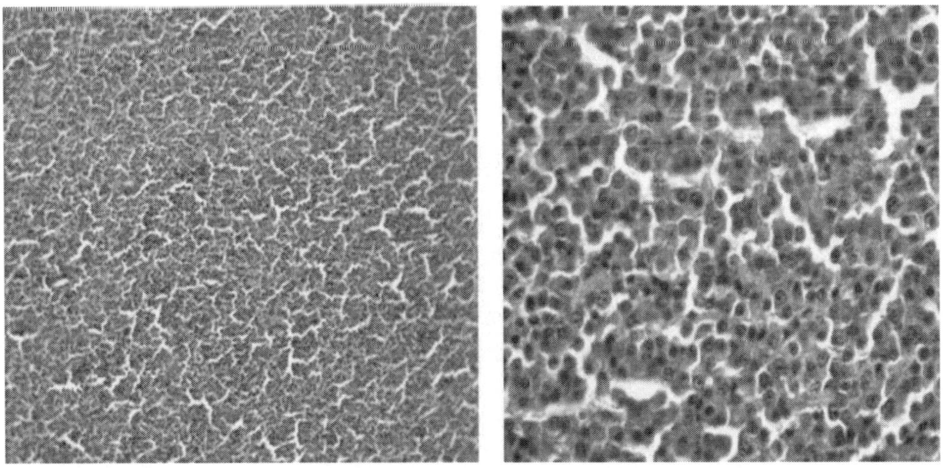

Figure 4-27. Plasmacytom: The cells are round or oval with an eccentric nucleus.

Treatment

- BMT (bone marrow transplant) in patients younger than 70 years.
- Current treatment regimen includes Steroids with one of the newer drugs (Lenolidamide, Thalidomide, or Bortzum). These drugs may resite bone marrow in the future.

- Melphalan or cyclophosphamide may need to be added to the above diet.
- Bisphosphonates are given to prevent bone resorption.
- Prognosis depends on cytogenetic findings, disease extent, patient age, and renal function.
- The overall median survival of patients with new treatments is 8 years.

Note

Areas where a lytic lesion may be more suspicious to be multiple myeloma than a metastasis includes:

- Distal clavicle
- Acromion
- Glenoid
- Olecranon
- Multiple discrete lesions in the skull

Types of Plasmacytomas

POEMS syndrome includes:

- polyneuropathy
- Organomegaly
- Endocrinopathy
- Monoclonal gammopathy
- Skin changes
- m> F
- in younger age than MM
- Also known as osteosclerotic myeloma, bone lesions can be single or multiple. 97% have an osteosclerotic component on radiographs, even if the component is small, or sclerotic, or limited to a thin sclerotic rim.
- Longer lifespan than myeloma.

Radiotherapy or chemotherapy depends on the size of the tumor.

MGUS

- Monoclonal gammopathy of undetermined significance.
- Increased monoclonal protein in the blood. This protein has to be less than 3 grams per deciliter.
- Bone marrow has less than 10% of clonal plasma cells.
- Has no dysfunction of other organs or bone lesions.
- 19% becomes aggressive form within 10 years.

Smoldering Myeloma

- Another name is asymptomatic myeloma.
- For diagnosis, it is necessary that: more than 10% of the clonal plasma involve the bone marrow or the serum M protein volume be more than 3 grams per deciliter.

- Has no dysfunction of other organs or bone lesions.
- Symptomatic multiple myeloma.
- Clonal plasma cells in the bone marrow with any amount usually associated with M protein in the serum.
- Existence of damage to internal organs including CRAB, which stands for:
- HyperCalcemia.
- Renal insufficiency.
- Anemia.
- Bone lesions.

Non-Secreted Mill

- More than 10% of clonal plasma cells are in the bone marrow.
- Less than half a milligram per deciliter of M component in serum.
- Have less than 200 mg in 24-hour light chain proteinuria.
- Free light chain is not measurable.

Single Bone Plasmacytoma SPB

- Single myeloma is the average age of 10 to 15 years younger than multiple myeloma.
- M = 2F.
- M protein in serum and urine is low or negative.
- Bone destruction is limited to one focus.
- Bone marrow has less than 10% of clonal plasma cells.
- Skeletal survey and MRI if normal.
- It does not have the dysfunction of other organs like what is observed in multiple myeloma.
- 60-50% of patients with SPB develop multiple forms after radiotherapy, usually within 4 years.
- Whole spine MRI or PET/CT of the whole body is necessary for the initial examination of multiple lesions until the diagnosis of SPB is reached.

Plasmacytoma Outside the Bone Marrow

- Component M is negligible in serum or urine.
- Tumors outside the bone marrow contain clonal plasma cells.
- Less than 5% of clonal plasma cells in the bone marrow.
- The skeletal survey is normal.
- Has no dysfunction of other organs or bone lesions.

BONE METASTASIS

General Points

- They are the most common bone tumors.
- The ratio of metastasis to primary bone tumor is 20: 1.

- Especially in patients older than 40 years and also in those who are young but have a known history of cancer, it should consider metastasis as the differential diagnosis of many lesions.
- Most metastases are in the spine or pelvis because blood flow is high in these areas.
- 75% of metastasis are lytic.
- After osteoarthritis, they are the most common cause of pathological fractures.
- Sclerotic lesions are caused by bone production by the tumor as well as by the host's repair mechanism.
- Although reactive ossification occurs in varying amounts in all metastasis, in severely destructive, rapidly growing lesions, there is insufficient opportunity to do so to the extent that the symptoms can be observed on radiographs.
  - 75% are lytic. It is when bone resorption takes precedence.
    - Kidney
    - Lung
    - Breast
    - Thyroid
    - Gastrointestinal tract
  - 15% are sclerotic. It is when bone formation predominates.
    - Prostate
    - Seminoma
    - Breast
    - Cervix
    - Ovarian
    - Bladder
    - Carcinoid
    - Osteosarcoma
  - 10% are a mixture of lytic and sclerotic.
    - Breast
    - Lung

Epidemiology

- Typically observed in people over the age of 40.
- 1.5 million new cases of cancer are diagnosed each year in the United States.
- 600,000 cancer deaths are reported annually in the United States. Two-thirds of these cases have bone metastases.
- 30% of patients with malignancy develop metastasis. This is much higher for the prostate and breast (85%).
- 60% of bone metastasis in men and 70% of women are related to prostate and breast, respectively.
- Most metastases develop within two years of the initial diagnosis of malignancy.
- Nuclear scans about 4 months earlier than radiographs can show bone metastasis.
- 80% of bone metastasis are following cancers of the breast, prostate, lung, kidney, and thyroid.

- Some malignancies rarely metastasize to the bone: tumors of the head and neck, pancreas, liver, esophagus, stomach, uterus, and ovaries are in this group.

Source

- Seed and soil theory of suitable seed in suitable soil.
- Radiated bone is not a good site to implant metastasis.
- Metastasis larger than 2 mm requires angiogenesis.
- Vascular endothelial growth factor.

Site

- Areas with high blood flow are more involved.
- The lumbar, thoracic, and cervical regions of the spine are involved, respectively.
- After the axillary bones, the femur and humerus are the most common sites for metastasis.
- Involvement of the vertebral pedicle is very beneficial for the lesion to be metastatic, although it occurs secondary to the involvement of the vertebral body.
- Involvement of the lesser trochanter, sternum, is also strongly in favor of lesion metastasis.
- 50% of Foot / Hand metastases
    - Lung
    - Breast
    - Renal
- In the prostate, they reach the pelvis and vertebrae through the Batson venous network.
- Gynecologic malignancies of the bladder and lungs can spread directly to the bones.

Clinical Signs

- Dull aching pain.
- Weight loss.
- It can be asymptomatic.
- Any Fx in a person with a history of cancer ß suspected of metastasis.

In 1981, Fidler Assessed the Risk of Fractures Based on Cortical Involvement

- In less than 50% of the cortex involvement, the risk of fracture is 2.3%.
- In 50 and 70% of the cortex involvement, the risk of fracture is 60%.
- In more than 75% of the cortex involvement, the risk of fracture is 80%.

In 1986, Harrington Proposed Prophylactic Fixation Based on the Size of the Lytic Lesion

- Involvement greater than 50% of the bone diameter.

- The diameter of the lesion is more than 2.5 cm.
- Persistent pain persists after radiotherapy.
- Persistent tumor growth persists after radiotherapy.

In 1989, Mirels Proposed a Criterion for Prophylactic Fixation Based on Four Variables

- The site of the lesion, the type of pain, the type of lesion, and the size of the lesion are four variables.
- Each of the above four variables can be awarded from 1 to 3 points.
- When the total score reaches 8 or more, prophylactic fixation is recommended.
- Another indication of prophylactic fixation of fractures is Avulsion fracture in lesser trochanter. This can quickly become a complete pre-trochanteric fracture and due to the complexity of the fx, the fixation will be harder (Figure 4-28) on the basis of articles about seventy percent of non-traumatic lesser trochanteric avulsion are related to metastasis and thirty percent Related to primary bone tumors including chondrosarcoma. In this case, a biopsy prior to prophylactic fixation of a lesser trochanter fracture is recommended so that if the malignant primary tumor is the diagnosis, wide resection is used instead of prophylactic fixation.

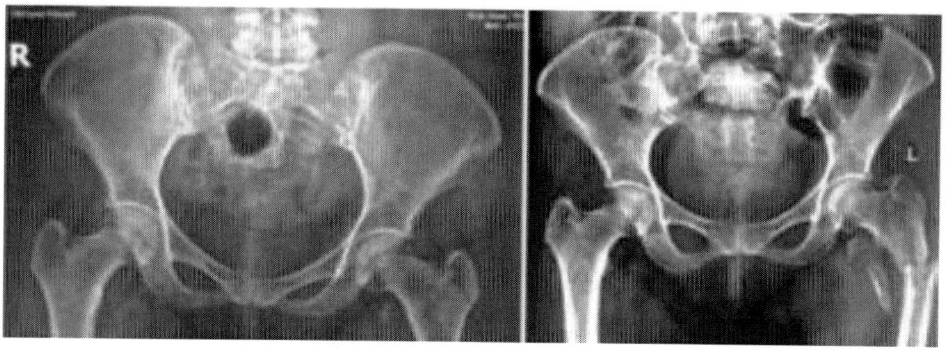

Figure 4-28. Avulsion fracture in the lesser trochanter in a 38-year-old woman that has been converted into a complete fracture after two weeks. The patient has metastatic breast carcinoma.

- Lesions of the femoral neck, humerus, and peritoneal area are highly prone to fractures.
- Near-joint lesions are diagnosed later because of the similarity of symptoms to DJD.
- Hyperemia is observed in lytic lesions due to increased bone resorption.
- Hypocalcemia is observed in prostatic blast metastasis.

Imaging

- They have no periosteal reaction.
- No sclerotic margin.
- Most metastases are intramedullary.
- Lytic appearance of soap scum dilator: observed in kidney or thyroid carcinoma.
- Dense multifocal sclerotic appearance without dilation: prostate

- Aggressive periosteal reaction with sunburst pattern: is rare, can be observed in prostate carcinoma, carcinoid tumor, and neuroblastoma.
- Internal calcification: Colon and thyroid carcinoma is observed.
- Metastasis to the cortex: Characteristics of breast and lung carcinoma.
- More than 30 to 50% of the thickness of the cortex has to be lost until noticeable changes are observed on the radiograph.
- In the pelvis, intestinal gas is difficult to diagnose and therefore CT is required.
- Skeletal survey is useful in kidney carcinoma and multiple myeloma because it may not be active on nuclear scan.

BS Bone Scan

- High sensitivity. More than 90% of metastasis have increased absorption.
- On average, 4 months before radiography can detect metastasis.
- Has little specificity. Non-neoplastic processes can increase absorption.
- Increased absorption in adjacent ribs is also a sign of fracture, not metastasis.
- In renal carcinoma, myeloma, thyroid carcinoma, and lymphoma may be negative.
- Metastasis may be in the form of cold spots.
- Super scan: When there is no activity in the kidneys and soft tissue and the radioactive drug is absorbed by metastatic bone (especially in the prostate). This mode gives the wrong view of normal scanning.
- Flare phenomenon: When there is an increase in the absorption of radioactive material following treatment:
    - Demonstrates a good response to treatment, because the lesion healing, ossification, and sclerosis may result in increased absorption of radioactive material into the lesion.
      It is observed in the first 3 months after treatment.
    - Has to improve within 3 to 6 months.
      It is more associated with chemotherapy and hormone therapy than radiotherapy

CT

- Indicates the extent of cortical damage.
- A difference of more than 20 Hansfield units between the right and left is considered abnormal.
- In treated metastasis, it indicates the severity of sclerosis and therefore a good response to treatment.

MRI

- The most sensitive means of diagnosis is to show metastatic disease
- Lytic: dark in T1 and bright in T2.
- Sclerotic: Dark on both sides.
- Target (Halo) sign A clear rim is observed in T2 around the lesion.

FDG PET

- Most solid tumors, especially those with a high metabolism (such as cancers of the skin, lung, colon, and lymphoma), are good for detecting bone metastasis.
- Is not very suitable for detection of tumors with low metabolism (prostate carcinoma, carcinoid, and bronchoalveolar carcinoma).
- It is better than a bone scan to find small lesions that do not have enough osteoblastic activity.
- Sclerotic metastasis show increased activity on the nuclear scan, but are negative due to lack of cellularity in FDG PET.
- Positive cases other than metastasis include fractures, degenerative changes, infection, Paget's disease, chemotherapy, and the use of G-CSF.

Treatment

- Fixation: if there is a risk of fracture.
- Bisphosphonate: Reduces pain and possibly reduces tumor volume by inhibiting osteoclasts. They have no effect on life expectancy.
- Nonsteroidal anti-inflammatory drugs (NSAIDs) and narcotics are prescribed to control pain.
- Hormone therapy is used for some breast and prostate cancers.
- Radiotherapy (external beam or Radionuclide method) with or without chemotherapy.
- In multiple metastases, the prognosis is poor. 5 months from the time of diagnosis until death for most primary cancers.

Differential Diagnosis

- Primary malignant neoplasms (sarcomas) are often larger than 10 cm, but most metastases are less than 4 cm. The woven components have a softer texture. The bone scan is negative multiple myeloma. Sarcomas have a more probiotic response than most metastasis (with the exception of prostate carcinoid, retinoblastoma, and neuroblastoma).
- Osteomyelitis
- Stress fracture
- Brown tumor

Cases That Are in Favor of Metastasis

- Multiple lesions
- Older age
- Existence of a lesion in the axial skeleton
- Metastasis is more likely to produce lesions of different sizes than multiple myeloma
- The periosteal component reacts less softly than the primary tumor

Carcinoma of Unknown Origin

- 2 to 6% of all malignancies.
- Has a poor prognosis. The average survival from the time of diagnosis is 11 months.
- In 25% of patients, even with an autopsy, the initial site is not discovered.

- Lesions that are not obviously benign have to be examined metastatically. This includes the following:
  - Tests include complete blood counts, urine tests, kidney, and liver function tests, stool occult blood tests, and PSA.
  - Imaging: CT scan of the chest, abdomen, pelvis, skeletal scan, mammography (some do not recommend mammography), and PET/CT.

Other

- The most common primary site of metastasis of unknown origin is in the kidneys and lungs.
- Distal lesions to the elbow and knee and bite lesions are mostly metastasis of primary lung origin.

Breast Metastasis

- It is generally the most common source of bone metastasis.
- Bone is the most common area of distant metastasis (non-lymph nodes) for breast cancer.
- Most breast cancer patients who die have metastasis.
- It is mostly lytic. Blastic lytic mixtures have the second prevalence, and the sclerotic type has the lowest prevalence.
- The axial skeleton and ribs are more involved.
- Proximal femur (neck and intertrochanteric) and cranial and dural metastasis are typical symptoms of advanced metastatic breast cancer.
- In 30% of patients with breast cancer, hypercalcemia occurs due to lytic lesions.

Prostate

- The most common source of bone metastasis in men.
- Bone metastasis is observed in 35-25% of patients with prostate cancer.
- 75% is sclerotic.
- Can give a sunburst positive reaction.
- Spread to the pelvis and spine through the Batson venous network
- Can give a view of the ivory vertebral body.
- Gives a broad appearance resembling Paget's disease.
- In bone metastasis, PSA is above 10 and often above 20.
- Can have a super-scan view during bone scan

Lung

- In 80% of the cases, it is lytic.
- The most common malignancy that occurs as single bone metastasis.
- Bilateral symmetrical metastasis to unusual areas, such as the patella, can be observed.
- Lung SCC can metastasize to the limbs.
- The ribs and chest wall can be infected by the direct spread of the tumor.
- The appendicular skeleton is often located in the cortex and may have abnormal radiographic images such as cortical lesions or periosteal lesions.

- It can give an apple-bite, cookie-bite view due to bone cortex involvement soft texture along with the component.

Kidney

- 90% are lytic.
- It is a tumor prototype that gives metastasis of unknown (often single) origin.
- It metastasizes to strange areas: skin, tongue, eyes, heart muscle, eye and breast.
- They can be septated, expansile and with a soft tissue mass.
- Most are hypervascular.
- Preoperative embolization significantly reduces bleeding and the need for RBC transfer.
- Metastasectomy A single metastasis increases life expectancy.
- Typically has a clear cell view.
- They can be dilated, have a septum, and have a soft tissue mass.
- Compared to other malignancies, it is more likely to be associated with pathological fractures because it is dilated and destructive in nature.

Thyroid

- Mostly lytic.
- After the lymph nodes in the neck, it metastasizes to the skeleton and lungs more than any other organ.
- Thyroid carcinoma is more prone to skeletal and lung metastases in younger people.
- Skeletal metastasis can be observed even 20 years or more after primary tumor treatment.
- The follicular type is more prone to bone metastasis.
- Can be expandable.
- May have calcification.
- It can pass through the joint space and include both sides of the joint.
- May be associated with thyrotoxicosis.
- Radioactive iodine can be used to treat primary thyroid disease and metastasis except in the anaplastic type.

Findings That Are in Favor of Metastatic Compression Fracture Than Being Osteoporotic Fracture

- The posterior margin of the body is convex.
- Abnormal signal in the pedicle or posterior elements
- Epidural mass
- Lack of low linear horizontal linear fractures at T1 and 2T
- Retro-pulsation of bone fragments to the posterior.
- Multiple fractures that are not adjacent.
- Adjacent disks are normal.

- Signal increase in diffusion weighted MRI and when the ADC values are less than the normal vertebral body.

Bone Metastasis in Children

- The most common are: Neuroblastoma, rhabdomyosarcoma, clear cell sarcoma of renal origin, T sarcoma, Ewing, s, osteosarcoma, leukemia, soft tissue sarcomas.
- Unlike adults, metastasis in children involve the appendicular skeleton more than the axial.
- Most metastasis are lytic.
- Metastasis from medulloblastoma, osteosarcoma, carcinoid tumors, and in some cases retinoblastoma can be sclerotic.

Neuroblastoma Metastasis

- Has a unique tendency to metastasize to the eyeball, jaw, and metaphysis of long bones.
- It is a prototype of pediatric malignancies that can occur as a single bone metastasis without the site of the primary tumor being known.
- Clinically and radiologically similar to osteomyelitis.
- In the pathology of small round cells gathered in the form of rosettes, it induces the appearance of Ewing sarcoma.

Kidney Clear Cell Metastasis

- It is the third neoplasm of pediatric kidney after Wilms and renal carcinoma.
- The peak age is two to three years old.
- Has a high tendency to metastasize to bone.
- Like neuroblastoma, it can occur as bone metastasis with the uncertain primary focus.

Rhabdomyosarcoma Metastasis

- The peak embryonic type is 3 to 5 years old.
- Alveolar type has a worse prognosis than embryonic.
- Their metastasis are typically lytic.
- The five-year lifespan of the embryonic type is 90% and the alveolar type is 70%.

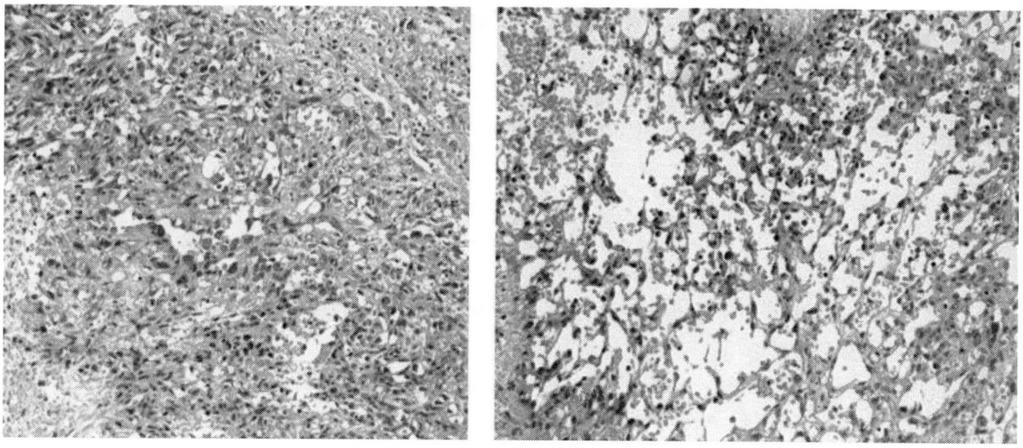

Figure 4-29. Angiosarcoma: This tumor is characterized by irregular vascular cyst-like spaces lined with atypical cells. These cells appear in the form of nests, ropes, or blades, and often spread papillary into the lumen of the vessel.

Chapter 5

TUMORS AND SOFT TISSUE LESIONS

LIPOMA

Definition

A benign adipose tissue tumor.

Epidemiology

- Lipomas are more common in middle-aged women.
- The average age is 48 years old.
- They can be multiple or symmetrical.
- Soft, round, mobile, painless, and slow-growing.
- The most common benign soft tissue tumor. It accounts for 10% of all soft tissue tumors and 16% of all benign soft tissue tumors.

Site

- Usually observed subcutaneous.
- The prevalence is common in the trunk, head and neck, lower limbs, buttocks, and upper limbs, respectively.
- Lipoma arborescens is most often found inside the knee. Involves the synovium and is associated with joint effusion

Lipoma inside of the joint is bright in T1 and dark in T2, and this is in contrast to the effusion inside the joint.

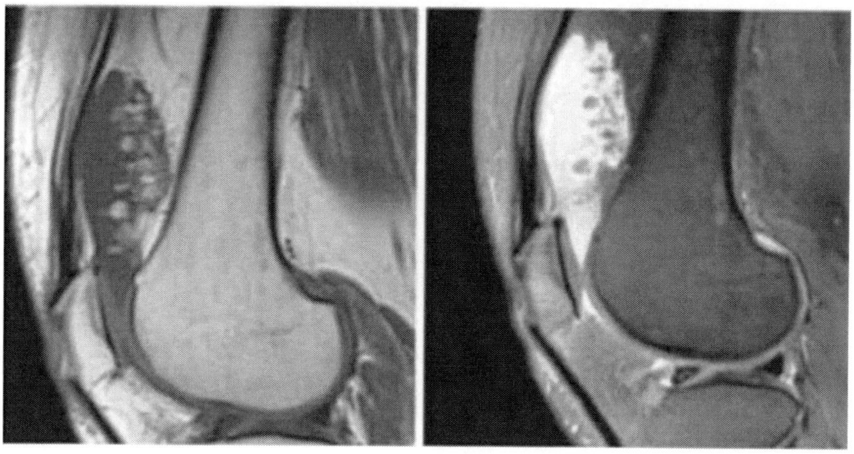

Figure 5-1. Lipoma arborescens. Left and right MRI T1 and T2 with fat suppressor, respectively.

Types of Lipomas

Dercum Disease

- Dominant autosomal disease with variable penetration in the form of infiltration of several subcutaneous lipoma.

Fetal Fat Cell Lipoma (Hibernoma)

- It is more common in postmenopausal women and in the pelvic girdle and thighs.
- Large mass of brown color and vacuolized tumor.
- The age peak is in the third and fourth decades. It is more common in men.
- They are typically subcutaneus (common in intracapsular and periscapular) and are commonly intramuscular in the limbs.
- The skin on the lesion is warmer due to the high flow of the tumor.

Angiolipoma

- In young adults, subcutaneous nodules are usually observed in the upper extremities.
- Rarely larger than 2 cm.
- In half of the cases it is bilateral.
- They are often painful, especially at the beginning of their development.
- Treatment is surgical resection.

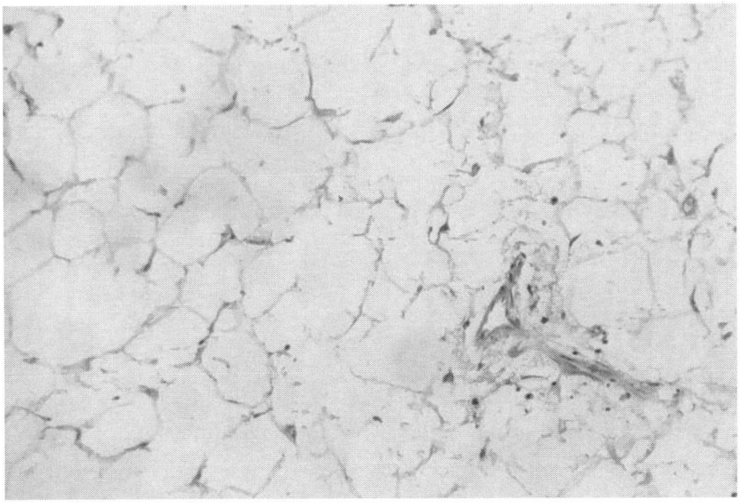

Figure 5-2. Lipoma.

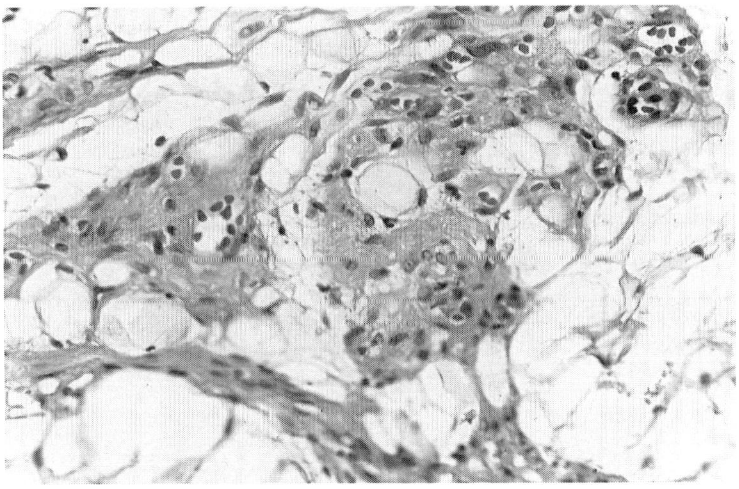

Figure 5-3. Angiolipoma: mature adipose tissue with thick-walled vessels, hyaline also is seen.

Angiomyolipoma

- It occurs in the kidneys or liver.
- Contains smooth muscle, fat and blood vessels.
- It is more common in women than men.
- Growth mass is usually slow but may also grow suddenly. The average size is 5 to 10 cm.
- Can cause abdominal pain, hematuria, bleeding inside the peritoneum.
- Doppler ultrasound shows vascular canals inside it.
- It is heterogeneous on MRI. It is slightly brighter than muscle on T1 and like fat on T2.

- It is not fat suppers.
- The treatment for complete removal of the tumor is extensive resection and recurrence is rare after complete removal.
- Sudden rupture is associated with bleeding and is one of the indications for arterial embolization.
- Angiomyolipoma in kidney is associated with tuberous sclerosis in the brain.

Myelolipoma

- Contains bone marrow elements found in the adrenal medulla.
- Occasionally observed in the presacral or mediastinum.
- If the diagnosis is confirmed, follow-up is recommended unless the lesion requires surgery due to its size.

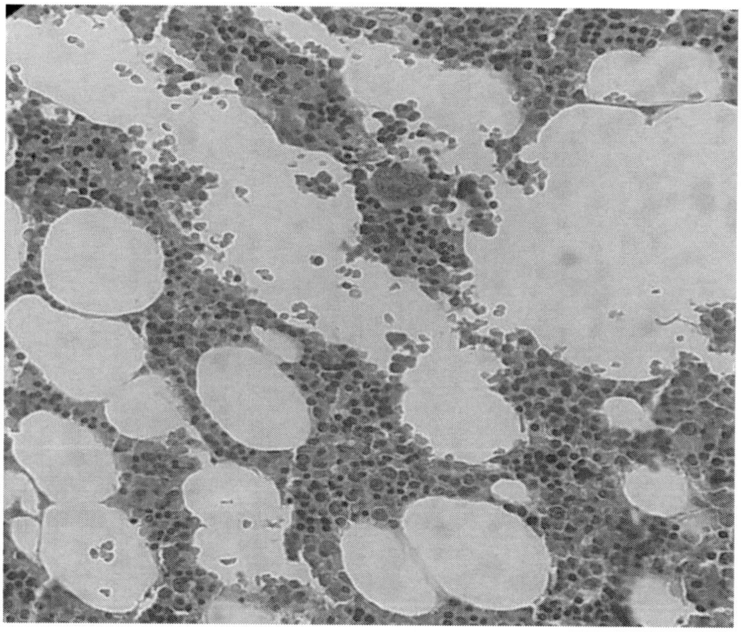

Figure 5-4. Myelolipoma: Mature adipose tissue with islands of hematopoietic cells.

Lipoblastomatosis

- Contains embryonal fat. It is observed in young children and infants. (Patients' age is usually less than 7 years old.) It is twice more common in boys than in girls.
- It is observed more in the trunk and limbs than the head and neck.
- It is composed of fetal white fat. Its average size is two to six centimeters.
- It has a lobular appearance.
- It has an excellent prognosis. Postoperative recurrence is reported to be about 14%.
- Many types are called Lipoblastomatosis.

Chondroid Lipoma

- It has cartilage inside the tumor.
- Differentiation: has to be differentiated from liposarcoma and myxoid chondrosarcoma.
- Spindle cell lipoma: Adult fat has been resited by fibroblasts. It is observed on the back of the neck in men aged 45 to 65 years.
- Intramuscular lipoma: In middle-aged adults, it is found in the form of a deep mass with slow growth, mostly in the thigh or trunk. In 10% of the cases it is non-infiltrative.

Treatment

- Follow-up/marginal resection

MRI

- The superficial type in T1 and T2 looks like subcutaneous fat.
- Deep inside the muscle, between muscles may infiltrate between muscle fibers and show striate view.
- Thin septa inside superficial or deep lipomas may be observed in FsT2. It is observed as an increase in signal.

Size

- Varies from 8 to 25 cm.
- It is 10 cm on average.
- GD: no gadolinium enhancement: even in septa, there is a slight increase in absorption.
- Hibernoma: serpentine vascular canals is observed with the slow velocity of blood flow that increases with Gd.
- It also increases the absorption of technetium due to the increase in metabolic activity

Lipoma Aborescens

- Often accompanied by joint effusion within synovium, hypertrophy of the frond-like areas is observed with a fat signal.

Lipoma on the Hand

- It is usually a painless mass that disrupts grasp.
- When it is around the MCP joints, it can lead to lateral deviation of the fingers.
- Compression of the ulnar or median nerves by lipoma can lead to impaired mobility or movement.
- Lipoma on hand often involves the digital nerves and is much larger than what is observed in adults. Therefore, conscious dissection is needed.

- Infiltrating lipomas, which occur in adults, are rare and without capsules and are benign, but are 60% more likely to recur and affect both intramuscular and intramuscular types.

Atypical Lipoma

- Necrotic, cystic, or calcification areas may occur within it.
- Most often, more than 75% of tumors are composed of fat. In liposarcoma, on the other hand, it is usually less than 75% fat.
- It is difficult to differentiate between low-grade liposarcoma and MRI.

Intravenous Lipofibroma

- It is benign and rare and usually affects the median nerve. The median nerve and digital branches are involved in eighty percent of the cases.
- It is common in the first three decades of life and is rarely observed after the age of thirty.
- Occurs with a mass on the surface of the palmar and wrist and the possibility of altered median nerve function.
- Fiber and adipose tissue infiltrate the nerve by infiltrating the epineurium.
- A biopsy may be needed for diagnosis.
- CTR or fasciotomy is recommended if there are signs of pressure on the nerve.
- Intravenous oxygenation is not recommended due to the possibility of fibrosis and nerve compression after surgery.
- Although deforming to malignancy is rare, pain that is unbearable necessitates surgery.
- In the field of digital nerves, surgery is performed as en bloc excision and nerve graft with acceptance
- The change in the sensation of the innervated area after the operation is observed by the patient in 30% macrodactyly.

Schwannoma

Definition

- A benign tumor originating from the nerve sheath.

Epidemiology

- The most common age of onset is 20 to 50 years old.

Site

- It originates from one of the major peripheral nerves.

Clinical Signs

- Painless mass is a common symptom in these patients.
- Referral pain can be observed in the area of the affected nerve, and tinnitus can be observed. These symptoms are very rare in other tumors.

Imaging

- A spindle-shaped mass in the affected nerve pathway that is dark in T1 and bright in T2. It is observed in the coronal or sagittal view.
- Split fat sign: The split fat around the tumor that is observed in the coronal or sagittal T1 (Figure 5-5).

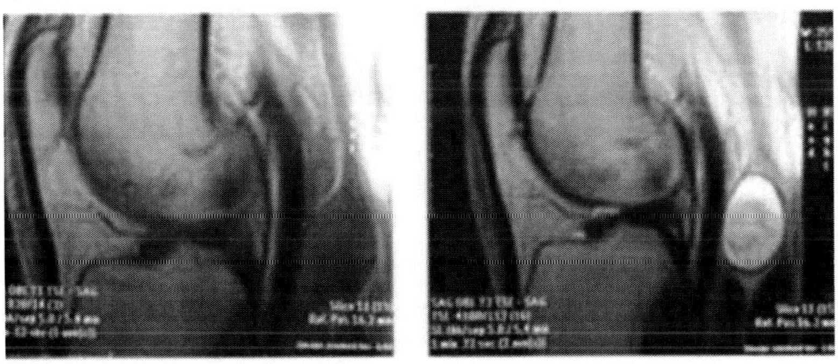

Figure 5-5. MRI of Schwannoma behind the knee. Left T1 and right. T2 tumor in the common peroneal nerve pathway.

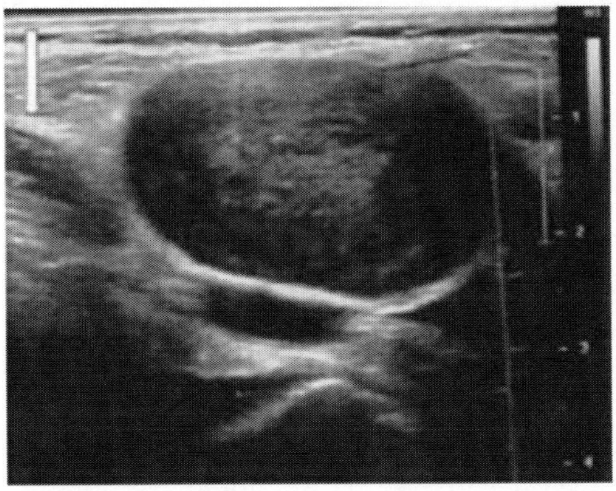

Figure 5-6. In this image, the spoon sign is observed, which is the schwannoma and the nerve originating from it (arrow.) The lesion is in the deep part of hyper echo (white color) and has the general appearance of a spoon.

- Target sign is observed in T2. It is a high signal in the periphery and a low signal in the center. To see this view, the MRI cut has to be perpendicular to the nerve pathway.
- In sonography, the spoon sign, the schwannoma, and the nerve originating from it are observed as a spoon (Figure 5-6).

Macroscopic Pathology

- It is observed as a spindle-shaped lesion along a nerve that has severed nerve fibers.

Microscopic Pathology

- It consists of two types of tissue.
- Antoni A consists of a dense accumulation of spindle-shaped cells.
- Antoni B is a myxomatous and degenerative tissue that is more common in tumor environments.
- Verocay bodies are found specifically in schwannoma. It consists of two rows of cells with a palisading core arrangement.
- S100 staining is positive, but not required for diagnosis.

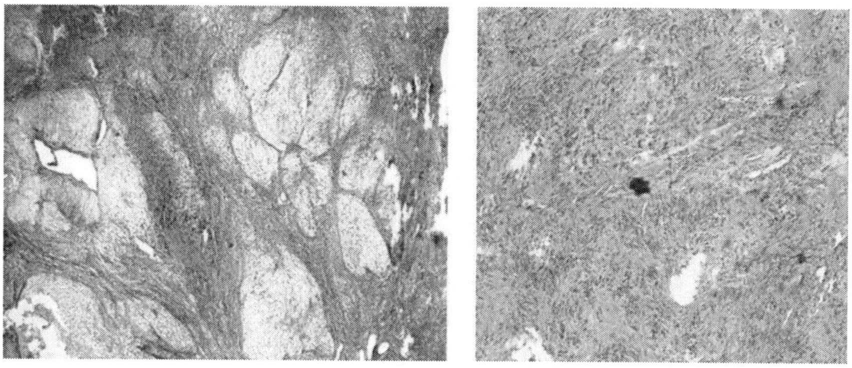

Figure 5-7. Schwannoma: Antoni A consists of a dense accumulation of spindle-shaped cells. Antoni B is a myxomatous and degenerative tissue that is more common in tumor environments.Verocay bodies are found specifically in schwannoma. It consists of two rows of cells with a palisading core arrangement.

Treatment

- Marginal resection with longitudinal incision on the epineurium.
- The tumor usually separates easily from the nerve without damaging nerve function.

NEUROFIBROMA

Definition

- They contain more collagen than Schwannoma.

Site

- It is found in smaller nerve trunks than in schwannomas.
- The nuclei of cells have a wavy shape.
- As the pain or size of the neurofibroma increases, transformation to malignancy has to be considered.

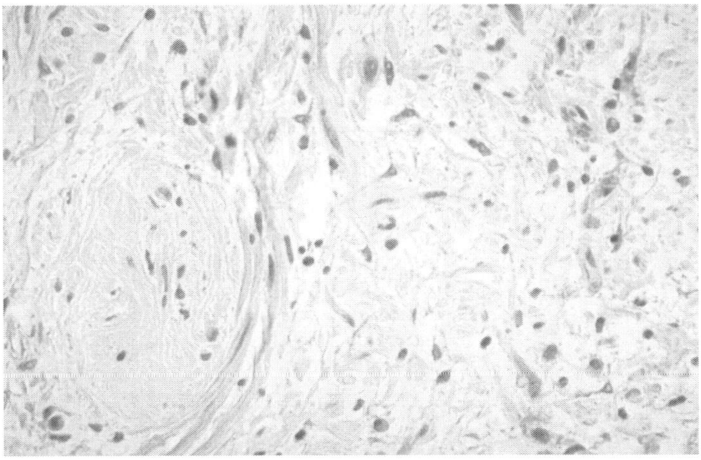

Figure 5-8. Neurofibroma: Spindle cells without pleomorphism, with wire-like collagen.

SYNOVIAL CHONDROMATOSIS

Definition

- A single joint disease is associated with synovial proliferation, in which cartilage metaplasia or cartilaginous ossification is observed.
- The synovial membrane engages the joint, bursa, or tendon sheath and leads to the formation of multiple cartilaginous nodules.
- Many nodules detach from the synovial membrane and float into the joint.
- Scattered synovium. The tendency to recur is high and can lead to detailed performance
- Severely disrupt.

Epidemiology

- It is rare.
- Age peak: fifth decade (decade) 1-7.
- M ÷ F = 2.

Site

- Large weight-bearing joints.
- There are 70% of the cases of involvement around the knee.
- 10% is bilateral, especially in those involving the knee, hip, elbow.
- The prevalence is observed in the knee, hip, and elbow, respectively.

Stages of the Disease

- Primary: with synovial chondrometaplasia, and without loose body
- Transitional: Active synovial disease with loose body
- Late: Loose bodies without synovium disease.

Clinical Signs

- Pain
- Inflamation
- Movement restrictions
- Symptoms may last for months to decades, averaging 5 years.

Radiography

- In 10% of the cases, calcification is not observed on radiography.
- Typically: Articular or pre-articular nodules with spot or ring calcification are observed.
- Over time, the level of mineralization increases.
- Eventually nodules, ring calcifications or ovoid skin with a lucent center are found.
- Bone erosion may be observed, which does not necessarily mean aggressive behavior. CT & MRI
- Especially MRI in the early stages of disease that mineralization is not enough yet.
- Punctate signal void: T1
- T2 indicates an increase in signal and may also show a multinodular view.
- Lesions involving smaller joints become more symptomatic in the early stages. At these stages, they have not yet been sufficiently mineralized to be observed on radiography.

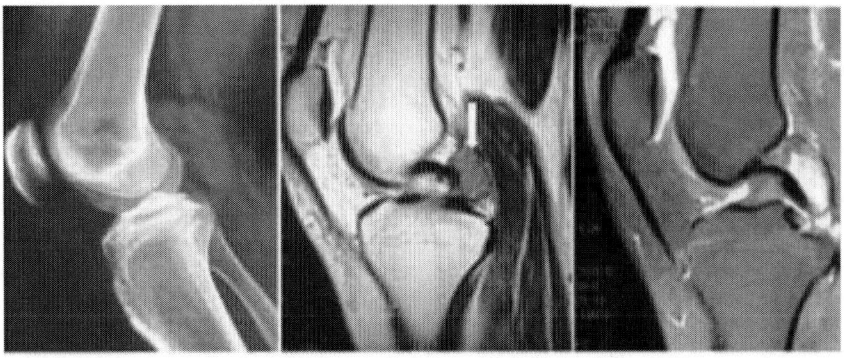

Figure 5-9. Synovial chondromatosis behind the posterior cruciate ligament in a 53-year-old man.

Macroscopic Pathology

- In advanced cases, the synovium is widely involved and is covered with cartilaginous multiple nodules.
- Nodules vary from less than one millimeter to more than one centimeter.
- Loose bodies also vary from one millimeter to 1-2 centimeters.
- Occasionally, adjacent bursae or tendons may be involved in prolonged cases.
- Types based on macroscopic pathology:
    - Diffuse: Multiple nodules that involve almost the entire synovium.
    - Localized: There is a distinct mass consisting of multiple nodules.
    - Outer joint involvement (bursa, tendon) is often observed at the same time as joint involvement rather than being separate. (It is rarely rarer than it is with joint involvement).

Microscopic Pathology

- Primary lesion: Hypercellular nodules contain chondroblastic cells with a small matrix.
- In Typic lesion, cartilage cells are loose.
- Early phases of cartilaginous metaplasia (primary lesion) is more common in smaller joints such as the hip or small joints of the hands and feet with a brief history of symptoms.nevertheless this is not a common condition and most patients have the long history of symptoms.
- Synovial chondroma: The presence of a nodule in the joint capsule. It is often observed in small joints such as the temporomandibular joint, and small peripheral joints.

Differential Diagnosis

- Chondrosarcoma is the most important differential diagnosis. Atypical cartilage cells are prominent.
- Secondary joint involvement with adjacent bone chondrosarcoma has to be ruled out in the first stage. This condition is especially common in the hip, where the chondrosarcoma of the pelvis or femur becomes infected.
- Rarely, synovial chondromatosis may develop within the bursa of an osteochondroma.

Treatment and Clinical Behavior

- Removal of involved bodies and synovial membranes or partial synovectomy by an open or arthroscopic method is sufficient in most cases. A complete synovectomy is not required.
- In some cases it is self-limited disease. After several years, the lesion becomes dormant, and only the symptoms of loose bodies inside the joint are active without the synovial disease.
- Extra-articular expansion and tendon involvement are not signs of aggressive aggression.
- Synovial chondromatosis has to be suspected in case of recurrent involvement with recurrent intermediate distance.

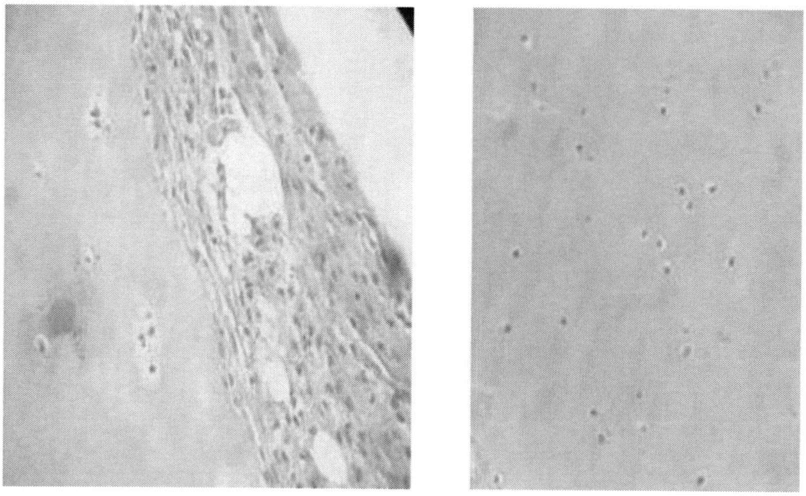

Figure 5-10. Synovial chondromatous. The cartilage cells in this view seem quite benign.

PVNS

Definition

- A proliferative fibrohistiocytic degenerative lesion consisting of villous and nodular protogens from.
  The synovial membrane is inside and outside the joint.

Types

- Local. Histologically it is the same as GCT of tendon sheath.
- Disseminated. The whole synovium is involved. The knee is the most common joint involved, but the hip, ankle, and wrist can also be involved. (Knee - 80% hip) 15%. The most common joint involved is the knee. The most common tenosynovium involvement is in the tendons of the hand.

Clinical Symptoms

- It usually occurs with pain and swelling of a single joint.
- Mechanical symptoms can be observed in intra-articular lesions.
- Movement restrictions.
- Joint blood effusion is common. The aspirated fluid is blood or brown in color.
- The duration of symptoms is relatively long. A few months to a few decades. Five years on average.
- Symptoms are intermittent or progressive.

Imaging

- Radiography is usually normal, but bone erosion can be observed, especially in hip involvement. This erosion can be severe and can lead to hip arthroplasty. In other joints, radiolucency can also be observed in the two joints in the epiphysis or metaphysis. There is fibrous tissue inside the bone lesions.
- May be associated with a detailed DJD and several sub-condyle cysts. Cysts are involved in both sides of the joint.
- MRI generally shows dark T1 & T2. In some cases the following changes can be observed:
  - Low signal: T1 is dark but not homogeneous and due to homogeneous sediments, it has dark dots (signal void).
  - T2: Areas with a high signal associated with edema or inflammation, and areas with a low signal associated with the presence of the most homozygous.

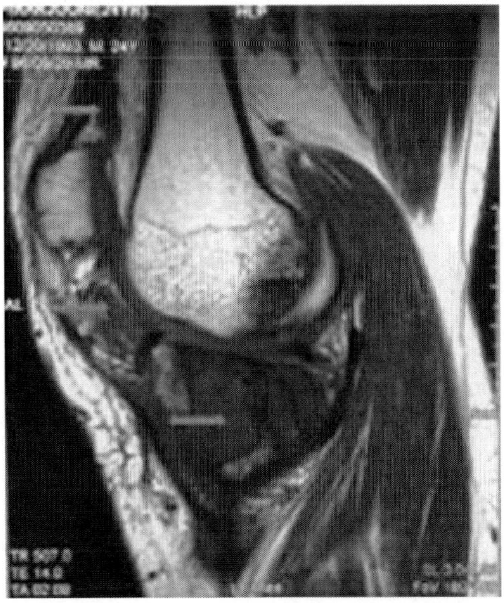

Figure 5-11. Pigmented venereal synovitis in the knee of a twenty-four year old man. Sagittal view of MRI 1. Arrows from top to bottom indicate lesions in the tibia, posterior to the patellar tendon, posteriorly to the patellar tendon, and posteriorly to the quadriceps.

Areas Involved

- Joints, bursae, tendons, adjacent fascia and ligament tissue, and a combination of all can get involved.
- There may be simultaneous intra-articular and extra-articular conflict.
- In general, the disease process is an inflammatory reaction process.

Incidences and Epidemiology

- Age peak: 3rd and 4th decades.
- M ÷ F = 1.

For Further Reading

Overall, when all PVNS & GCT cases of tendon sheath are examined together, the affected areas are in the following order:

- Fingers 60%
- Knee 30%
- Toes 10%

Macroscopic Pathology

- In the diffuse type, all or most of the synovium is involved.
- Papillary projections appear brown or tan (due to hemosiderin).
- The joint capsule is thickened.
- Yellow areas are due to lipid deposition in foamy histiocytes.
- The margin of the lesion that mixes with the surrounding tissue is blurred.
- Joint cartilage and adjacent bone may erode.

Microscopic Pathology

- Collectively fibrohistiocytic proliferations.
- Homocysteine deposition is noticeable.
- Foamy histiocytes are observed singly or in clusters.
- Histiocytes and giant multinucleated cells are also available.

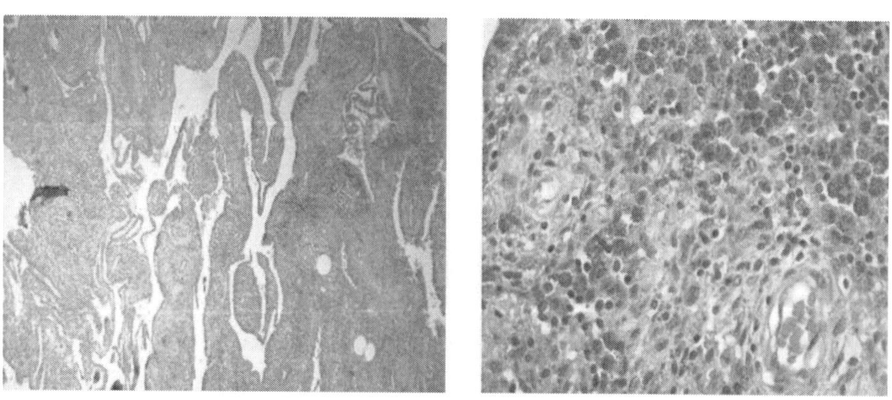

Figure 5-12. PVNS: Papillary and villous pattern show the proliferation of polygonal cells with multinucleated giant cells and hemosiderin-laden macrophages.

Differential Diagnosis

- Rheumatoid arthritis: Has villous synovial changes, but there is plasma cell infiltration that is not a PVNS specimen.
- Post-traumatic synovitis also has villous changes, but cell infiltration observed in PVNS is not present in the traumatic type of synovitis.
- Hemarthrosis in hemophilia: Usually no hemosiderin deposition.
- Epithelioid sarcoma: may be mistaken, especially with nodular extra-articular type. PVNS does not have epithelial markers does not have future mitosis and geographic necrosis that mimics rheumatoid nodules is also absent. Joint hemangiomas and chronic joint infections are also considered as a differential diagnosis.

Treatment and Clinical Behavior

- Frequent and locally aggressive recurrences are a feature of PVNS.
- Adjacent bone erosion and severe joint dysfunction can occur.
- Treatment involves the removal of the synovium. In local cases, it involves marginal resection and in diffuse cases, it includes complete synovectomy.
- The recurrence rate is about 30 to 50% even with a complete synovectomy.
- Severe involvement of the synovium and adjacent bone requires a prosthesis.
- Radiotherapy is effective in preventing further joint damage and reducing the risk of recurrence. A low dose is used.
- In very rare cases, it turns into spindle cell malignancy after many recurrences.

Soft-Tissue Vascular Tumors

General

- There are benign lesions that bear a strong resemblance to normal blood vessels. It is difficult to differentiate hamartomas and malformations and tumors.
- Most of them are superficial.
- Capillary hemangioma is the most common type of hemangioma.
- Mostly tend to involve the head and neck.
- They can affect internal organs such as the liver
- They are very common. They make up 7% of benign tumors.
- This tumor is more common in infancy and childhood.
- M> F for superficial hemangiomas
- Can resize with pregnancy and menstruation. The endothelial cells of these tumors may respond to hormones.

Types

- Strawberry
  - It occurs at birth or shortly thereafter.

- Bold red.
- In the first few months of life may grow rapidly.
- After a while, it stops growing and usually regresses.
- Rarely needs surgery.
- Port wine:
  - Often observed on the face, neck, and upper torso.
  - Occurs at birth or shortly thereafter
  - Its growth is proportional to the growth of the child.
  - Does not disappear by itself.
  - Surgery is very difficult.

Intramuscular Hemangioma

- Most of the lower extremities, especially the thigh muscles, are involved.
- Young people are more involved. 80 to 90% of patients are under 30 years old.
- It can be painful. Pain during muscle activity or hanging limbs.
- Pain is more common in hemangiomas that are located in the long and narrow muscles, such as sartorius.
- It is the most common type of deep hemangioma.
- Discoloration of the skin on the face, visible pulse, or audible bruit: all are very rare.

Synovial Hemangiomas

- Capsules, soft tissue around the joints, or tendon sheets may become involved.
- The peak age is the second decade. Usually sympatheticThey start in childhood. Lesions are diagnosed in young people.
- The knees then the elbows are the most commonly involved joints.
- In the extra-joint type, the tendons, wrists and hands are involved.
- Symptoms include vague pain, limited mobility, and a palpable mass that heals as the small muscle is lifted.
- Peripheral nerve hemangiomas.
- Mostly observed under 40 years old.
- The trigeminal, ulnar, median, posterior tibial, and peroneal nerves are more commonly involved.
- Pain is common.
- Numbness of the innervated area with the nerve involved may exist.
- Muscle atrophy may exist.
- It also causes carpal tunnel syndrome.
- Mostly cavernous.
- Intrafascicular dissection with a microscope is the best surgical procedure
- Tumor glomus: will be described at the end of the season.

Imaging

- Soft tissue mass.
- Phlebolith.
- Serpentine view observed on MRI (Figure 5-13).
- Arteriography shows a vascular lesion with premature escape of the contrast material to the venous system.
- Moreover, in arteriography, the arteries are sited parallel to each other in a linear pattern.
- The above view is due to the growth of arteries between muscle fascicles and confirms the benignity of vascular lesions.
- When using gadolinium, they have a sharp increase in contrast.

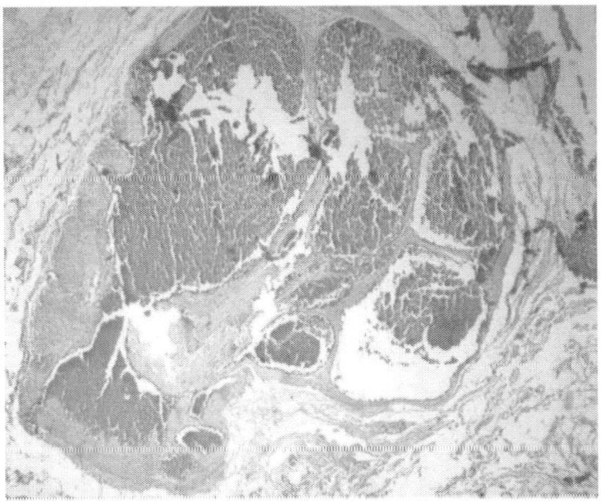

Figure 5-13. Intramuscular hemangioma.

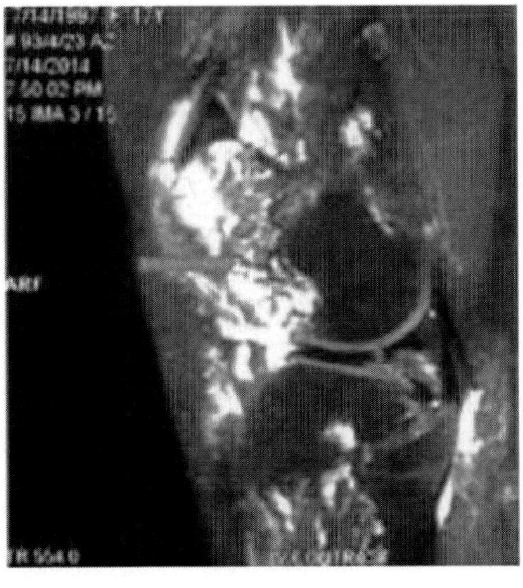

Figure 5-14. View of serpentine (arrow) in knee joint hemangiomas.

Microscopic Pathology

- Capillary or a mixture of capillaries - cavernous.

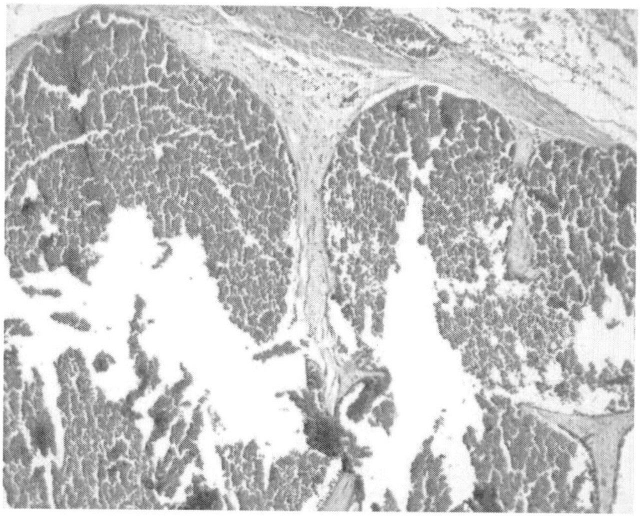

Figure 5-15. Intramuscular hemangioma.

Treatment and Clinical Behavior

- Postoperative recurrence is reported from 18% to more than 50%.
- Previous lesion embolization helps with surgery.
- Tumor recurrence is associated with insufficient primary excision.

Glomus Tumor

Definition

- It is a neoplasm that resembles a normal glomus body.
- It is classified as a perivascular tumor.

Epidemiology

- It is rare.
- It is most often diagnosed in 20 to 40 years. However, the symptoms have been present for several years before the diagnosis.
- M = F in general.
- M = 1/3 F in lesions under the nail.
- In neurofibromatosis, multiple glomerular tumors under the nail have been reported.

Common Site

- The most common site is under the nail.
- Palms, wrists, forearms and feet are the next most common.
- It is generally located deep in the derm or under the skin of the upper or lower limbs.

Clinical Signs

- The most common complaint is pain attacks that spread from the lesion.
- Pain episodes can occur spontaneously due to thermal changes (especially to the cold) as well as the touch of the lesion.
- Atrophy, hyperesthesia, and osteoporosis of the affected area, as well as Horner syndrome, may be associated with pain.
- The nail becomes grooved or discolored.
- Pain is caused by the release of substance P.

Imaging

- Small scalloped lytic defect with sclerotic margin at the terminal phalanx (Figure 5-16).
- In the bony type which is less common, it is observed as a lytic lesion smaller than one centimeter with a distinct margin without sclerosis, similar to osteoid osteoma.

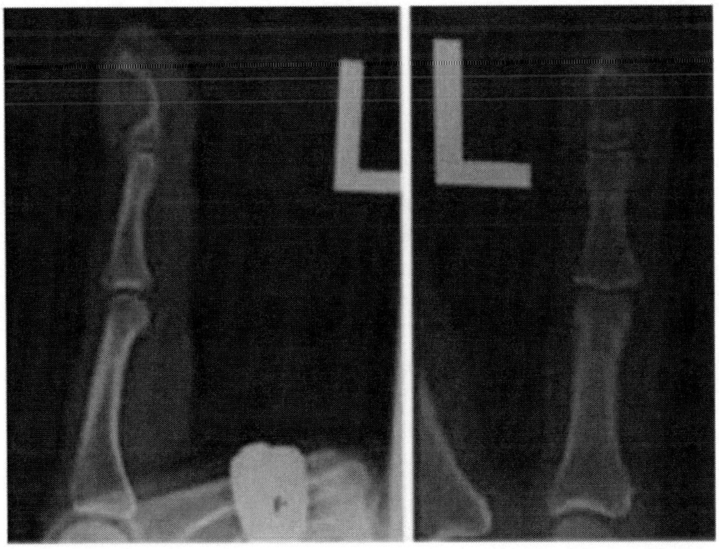

Figure 5-16. Plain radiograph of the left glomus tumors of the index phalanx. The lesion is usually observed as a radiolucent depression with a distinct sclerotic margin in the distal dorsal part of the phalanx.

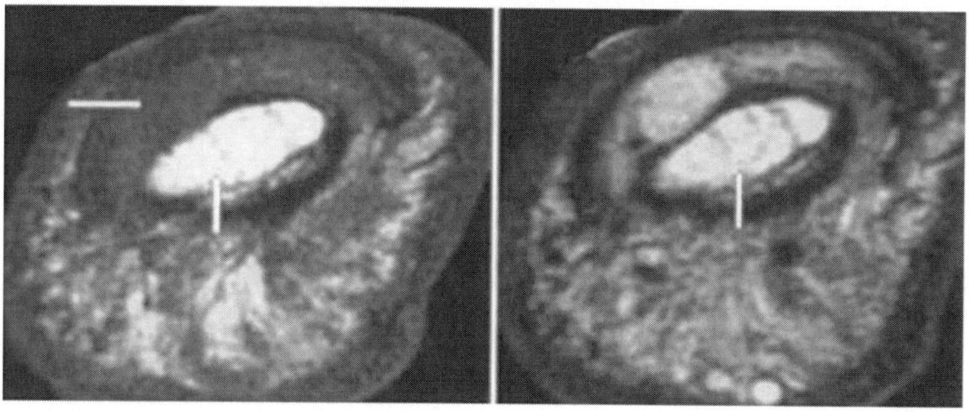

Figure 5-17. Glomus tumor MRI. Left and right T1 and T2 with fat suppressor, respectively. The vertical arrows represent the distal phalanx, and the horizontal arrows represent the tumor, which is observed at T1 as a low signal.

Macroscopic Pathology

- Small, reddish-blue nodules less than 1 cm in size that can be detected immediately on physical examination.
- A change in the color of the nail bed or the protrusion of the nail are symptoms that help to diagnose a lesion under the nail that is more difficult to diagnose.

Microscopic Pathology

- It is a lesion with a distinct margin, including dense arteries that are covered by endothelial cells.
- The arteries are surrounded by columns or nests of glomus cells with the appearance of a teloid in a hyaline or stromal stroma.
- Depending on the size of the glomerulus cells, the tumor may have a vascular or epithelial appearance.
- The glomus cell has a specific shape that helps differentiate the glomus tumor from other tumors.
- The shape of the glomus cell is regular and round with a central round punched out inside the cytoplasm of eosinophils.
- PAS staining of the intracellular matrix reveals the appearance of chicken wire, and therefore the margins of those that may be indistinguishable from hematoxylin staining are identified.

Treatment

- Most are benign and are treated with simple excision.
- Recurrence with the above method is only 5%.

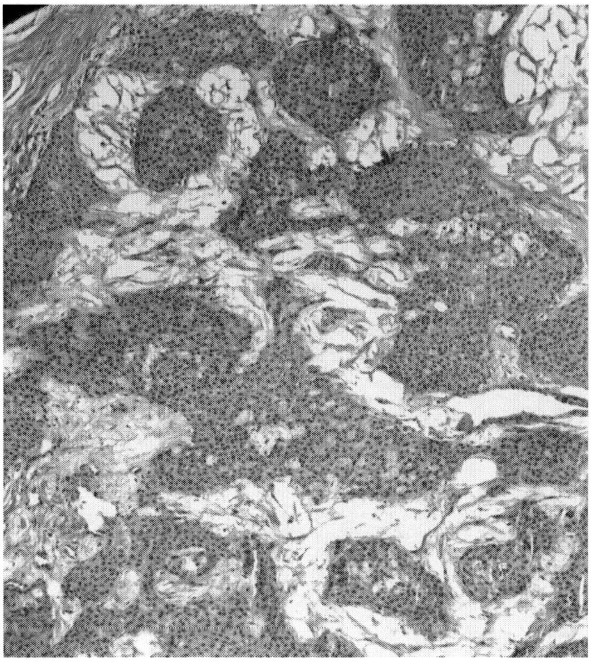

Figure 5-18. Glomus tumor: the glomerular cells around the arteries.

Note

- The function of the glomus body is to regulate temperature and blood pressure. In fact, it is a shunt.
- Glomus cells are round or oval perivascular muscle cells.
- Myelin-free nerves are responsible for transmitting pain.
- Love test: Creating severe pain by applying direct pressure to a tumor with a small, stiff body, such as a self-propelled tip.
- 75% are in hand.
- 25 to 65% are located under the nail.

STRAWBERRY HEMANGIOMA

Clinical Signs

- It is a flat red lesion similar to a birthmark, which is intensified by the baby crying.
- Highlights over time and finds the appearance of a strawberry nevus.
- Deeper lesions may be difficult to detect due to slight discoloration.
- They are not congenital but appear within the first few weeks of life.
- Grow rapidly within a few months.
- They reach the largest size in 6 to 12 months.
- Regress within a few years.
- The regression of the lesion is characterized by a change in the color of the skin towards it and its wrinkling.

75% to 90% regress by age 7, leaving a pigmented scar.

Pathology

- It is a nodular multiform mass fed by an arteriole.
- Primary lesions have plump endothelial cells.
- Mature lesions become more flattened endothelium similar to adult capillary hemangiomas. The pubic process progresses from periphery to the center.
- In retrograde lesions, fibrosis is observed between cells. The regression mechanism is cellular apoptosis.

Treatment

- Masterful neglect treatment is recommended to be done .only follow up should be done.
- Large life-threatening lesions that press on important organs (airways): Treatment with systemic steroids or interferon α.
- The treatment period is long. Interferon α can give spastic depletion.

Pyogenic Granuloma

- It is a type of polypoid capillary hemangioma.
- It is a reactive neoplasm or hyperplasia.
- It has the same prevalence in all decades of life.
- 60% mucosal levels.
- 40% skin.
- Prevalence: gums, fingers, lips, face, tongue.
- Within a few weeks to a few months, the tumor rapidly reaches its maximum size, which is a few millimeters to several centimeters.
- The polypoid lesion is brittle with a reddish-purple color that bleeds easily and is commonly sore.
- Baseless varieties are usually recurrent lesions.
- 1/3 cases occur following trauma.
- They can also occur during pregnancy and during retinoid treatment.
- They are an exophytic growth that attaches to the skin with a stem. Normal tissue is sometimes observed as a neck around the tumor stem.
- The epithelium on the lesion is atrophic, flat, or injured.
- The epithelium adjacent to the lesion is hyperkeratotic or acanthotic.
- The lesion is lobular. Each lip has an arteriole and a number of small capillaries.
- Acute and chronic inflammatory cells have spread throughout the lesion. Especially at the lesion level.

- In retrograde lesions, stromal fibrosis and fibrosis around the arteries are observed.
- Differential diagnosis: Malignant vascular tumors. In malignant tumors, the vascular spaces are irregular and the margin of the tumor is indistinct. Areas with spindle-shaped cells that surround cleft vascular spaces are found in malignant vascular tumors such as Kaposi's sarcoma. It has to be noted that the above cases have been observed in the deep or central areas of malignant tumors, so a biopsy of the superficial areas of these tumors may not be malignant.
- Sixteen percent have a recurrence after surgery.
- Recurrence is observed as a single nodule or satellite nodules around the site of a previous lesion.
- Recurrence is observed as satellite lesions, especially in the trunk, around the scapula, and the epithelium.
- It is usually healthy on satellite lesions.
- Recurrence was associated with incomplete removal of the tumor.
- Recurrence of lesions is treated by removing them again and sometimes they go away on their own.
- Recurrent lesions can be treated with catheter, sclerotherapy or laser curettage.

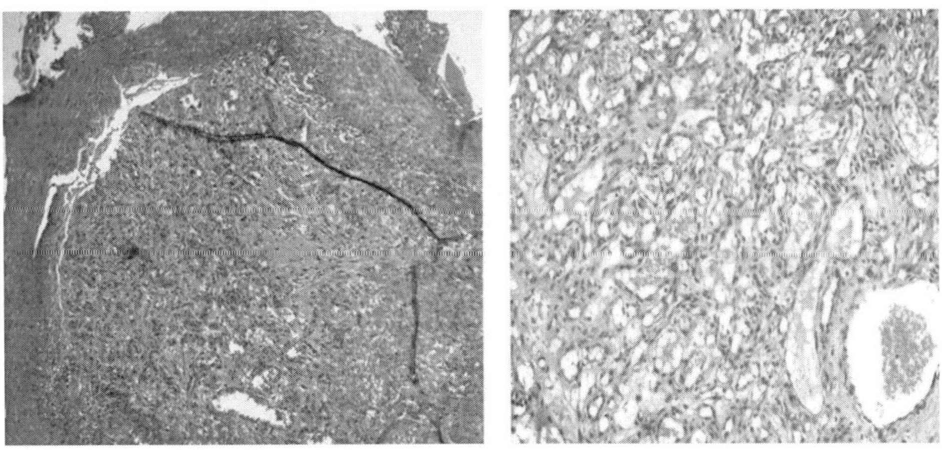

Figure 5-19. Pyogenic granuloma: lobular pattern of vascular proliferation.

Pyogenic Granuloma of Pregnancy

- Granuloma gravidarum is another name for it.
- Occurs at the level of the gums in 1% of pregnancies.
- They start from the interdental area of the gums and develop rapidly during the first trimester of pregnancy.
- They show significant regressions after delivery, although many may remain as small nodules until they regrow in subsequent pregnancies.
- The growth dependence of these lesions on hormones is evident that they are neoplastic (they do not have autonomic growth).

Senile Angioma

- Other names: Cherry angioma and Campbell de Morgan Spots.
- It is very common in adults, especially the elderly.
- Trunk and limbs. With age, their number increases.
- Red papules with pale surroundings a few millimeters in size.
- It is superficial in the dermis.
- They are composed of dilated capillaries with thin walls.
- They are associated with mild atrophy of the upper skin.

Cavernous Hemangiomas

- It is rarer than the capillary type.
- They have the highest prevalence in childhood.
- They are more common in the upper body.
- They are larger.
- They have a more indistinct margin.
- More commonly, they affect deep buildings.
- Do not tend to regress.
- They may be destroyed by pressure on nearby buildings. Therefore, unlike capillary hemangiomas, they often require surgery.
- The surface is swollen as a mass. They are blue with an irregular surface.
- Deeper lesions may not cause visible discoloration.
- In plain radiography, water-density masses are localized or diffuse.
- Calcifications are common in various forms. The type of phleboliths is both more common and more specific than calcification.
- Calcifications, both phlebolithic and amorphous, occur as a result of secondary dystrophic calcification organized into clots.
- It is a large, dilated blood vessel covered with a broad epithelium.
- The vessels are arranged in a lobular or irregular manner.

Cavernous Hemangioma-Related Syndromes

Kasabach-Merrit Syndrome

- Large hemangiomas with thrombocytopenic purpura. Most hemangiomas are large and occur on the limbs.
- Typically occurs in infancy.
- As the tumor grows rapidly, purpura can also be observed.
- Multiple skin ecchymosis and petechiae form due to intravascular coagulation and entrapment of platelets within the tumor.
- If left untreated, 30% of patients die from bleeding and infection.

- Treatment includes steroids, radiotherapy or interferon a 2 - α.
- Surgery is often impossible due to the hematological condition as well as the large size of the tumor.

Maffucci Syndrome

- Rare mesodermal dysplasia includes multiple hemangiomas and enchondromas.
- Hemangiomas are cavernous and commonly occur at birth.
- Lymphangioma and phlebectasia may also be present.
- Enchondromas form after hemangiomas.
- Between 20 and 100% of the cases chondrosarcoma and rarely angiosarcoma occur.
- Blue rubber bleb nevus
- Skin lesions are bluish in color with a plastic consistency that fades with compression and leaves a wrinkled skin that is then compressed and removed.
- There may be hyperhidrosis on the lesions.
- Most patients with hemangiomas have gastrointestinal tract and usually the small intestine. Bleeding from these hemangiomas is common and adds chronic anemia to the clinical picture.
- Treatment includes resection of intestinal bleeding lesions.

LYMPHANGIOMA

Definition

- It is difficult to differentiate them as true neoplasms, hamartomas, or lymphangiectasias.
- They are all benign.

Epidemiology

- Most often show up in childhood.
- M = F or M> F (quantitative).

Site

- Most are located in the head and neck and axilla, i.e., in the lymph nodes of the primary sacs.

Clinical Signs

- They are rarer than hemangiomas.
- 50 to 60 percent are present at birth.
- 90% occur by the end of the second year.
- They have been observed in association with hemangiomas in Maffucci syndrome.
- A wavy soft tissue mass that can remain constant, grow and shrink, or continue to grow.
- In cases following rapid URI, which causes obstruction of the draining lymph nodes, rapid growth occurs.
- Lymphangioma (cystic hygroma) can also be detected by ultrasound inside the uterus. It is associated with hydrops phthalic or Turner syndrome and has a high mortality rate.
- Tend to recur after resection.
- They have no potential for malignancy. Aggressive surgery has to be avoided, otherwise scarring will be a problem.

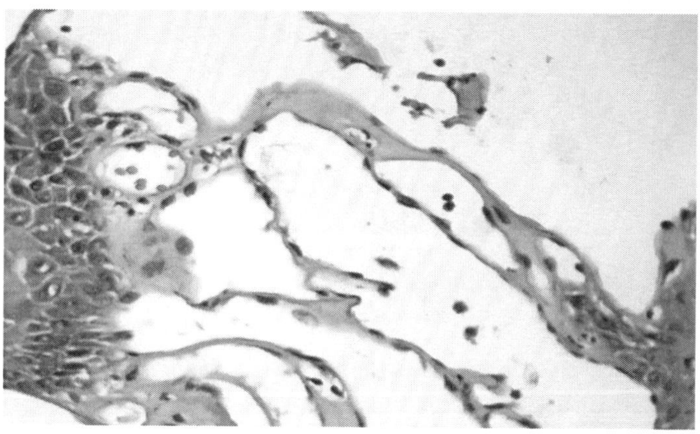

Figure 5-20. Lymphangioma.

FIBROMATOSIS

Site

- Shoulder girdle
- Pelvic girdle
- Thigh

Epidemiology

- F> M.
- The most common age is puberty up to 40 years old with a peak age of 25-35 years.

Clinical Signs

- Deep mass with indistinct margin, firm.
- It is painless or has little pain.
- Has a gradual growth.
- Decreased range of motion of adjacent joints may occur.
- Neurological symptoms, including drowsiness, stabbing/shooting pain, or motor weakness, can be caused by nerve compression.
- Soft tissue mass.
- Erosion or concussion of the adjacent bone can be observed due to the pressure of the tumor.
- A study shows that 80% of patients are associated with multiple involvement of the bones adjacent to the mandible, chest, or long bones.

Anatomical site of the extra-abdominal type

- Shoulder girdle
- Chest wall and back
- Thigh
- Head and neck
- Shoulder: the deltoid, scapula, suprascapular cavity, or posterior triangle are more affected. In this area, complete excision is difficult or even impossible.
- Pelvic girdle: Covers mainly the gluteal muscles but involves the quadriceps muscle and the popliteal muscles in the thigh.
- Hands and feet are rarely involved.
- Clinically, head and neck involvement is more severe than other areas of extra abdominal fibromatosis.

Multicentric Fibromatosis

- 5%.
- Typically involve an anatomical area.
- In most cases, the second growth proximal to the first lesion occurs.

Imaging

- At T1 it has a signal equal or lower than the muscles. It has a medium signal in T2.

Macroscopic Pathology

- The tumor is always confined to the muscles or aponeurosis of the upper fascia.
- Occasionally, it covers the periosteal lesion and leads to bone erosion. As a result, it becomes similar to the desmoplastic fibroma.
- Size: Most often 10 - 5 cm in the largest dimension.

- The tumor is hard and during cutting, a feeling of gritty is created.
- On the cutting surface, the glossy white appearance is similar to that of scar tissue with rough trabeculae. As a result, it is difficult to differentiate it from cases recurring from the scar tissue.

Microscopic Pathology

- Has an indeterminate margin.
- Specifically, the surrounding tissue usually infiltrates the striated muscle.
- Slender, spindle, and elongated cells with uniform appearance with large amounts of collagen
- Separated and cell-to-cell contact is negligible. There is no hyperchromia.
- The nuclei are small, pale, and have a definite margin.
- Collagen cells and fibers are sometimes arranged in sweeping bundles. Extensive hyalinization may occur and obscure the basal pattern of the lesion.
- At the periphery of the lesion, the tumor has infiltrated the muscle tissue. The rest of the striated muscle cells are similar to Giant's multinucleated cells.
- Microscopic hemorrhage and focal accumulation of lymphocytes are common.

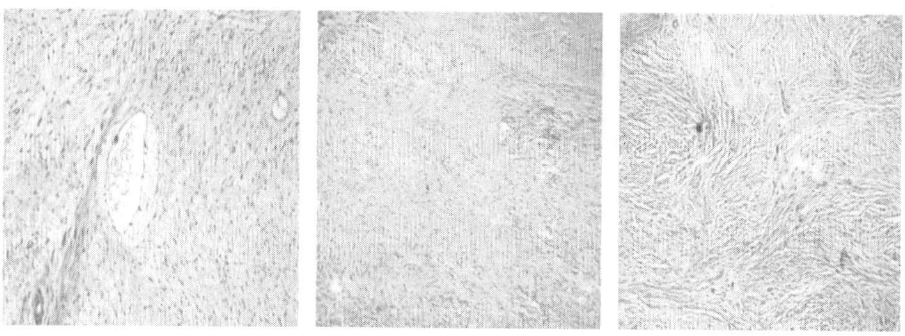

Figure 5-21. Fibromatosis: Classic fascicular view. This view shows the collagen stroma containing tall fibroblast fascicles. Small vessels are a clear indication of this tumor.

Differential Diagnosis

- Fibrosarcoma:
  - They have a herringbone-like appearance.
  - Cellularity is more uniform.
  - Cells overlap, and less collagen separates them.
  - The nuclei are more hyperchromatic and atypical and have more prominent nuclei.
  - More than one mitosis per 10 HPF is in favor of Fibrosarcoma.
  - A small biopsy specimen may lead to a misdiagnosis of these two, ie fibrosarcoma fibromatosis, and vice versa.
  - Reactive fibroblastic proliferation.
  - Occurs Following trauma, a minor muscle rupture or intramuscular injection.
  - Low magnification helps more differentiation: In reactive proliferation, there is focal bleeding or focal hemosiderin, which is often along the arteries.
  - Infiltrative growth pattern is in favor of fibrosarcoma.

Desmoplastic Fibroma

- It is very similar to fibromatosis, especially when it protrudes from the bone through a thin or enlarged cortex.
- This lesion is more common in the metaphysis/diaphysis of long bones or in the jaw.

Myxoma

- This is especially true with endo needle biopsy.
- Myxoma is small and the cells are separated by an abundant myxoid matrix.
- In fibromatosis, it has more interstitial cells and collagen.

Other

- Transformation of fibromatosis to fibrosarcoma is very rare.

Clinical Behavior

- Contrary to the benign microscopic appearance, the clinical behavior of the tumor is aggressive.
- No metastasis, usually recurrent.
- It can be fatal by squeezing vital organs, such as at the base of the neck or inside the abdomen.
- Recurrence of 19 to 77% of variables is reported and has an average recurrence of 40%.

Favorable Factors for Recurrence

- Large tumor size.
- Inadequate initial excision.
- Spontaneous regression has also been reported.

Treatment

- Most often wide excision unless there is a risk of severe functional loss in the patient. In that case, resection is performed to a lesser extent.
- Amputation if:
  - Frequent recurrence and non-response to adjuvant treatment.
  - The size of the tumor does not suggest another choice.

Radiotherapy

- For incompletely removed tumors.

Other

- Endocrine factors, such as abdominal fibromatosis, may also affect the type of extra-abdominal.
- Trauma can be a trigger.
- Hodgkin's report of fibromatosis following radiotherapy is available.

Focal Myositis

Definition

- A benign inflammatory tumor is a self-limiting benign inflammatory tumor

Epidemiology

- Observed in a wide age range.
- The average age is 36 years.

Common Site

- It is mostly observed in the limbs, especially the lower ones.
- Typically one muscle is involved.

Clinical Signs

- Has a rapid emergence and growth.
- It is usually asymptomatic except for the existing swelling.

Weakness is uncommon, and joint involvement is not observed.

Imaging

- Has a heterogeneous appearance.
- In T1 it is a low signal and in T2 it is a high signal.

The surrounding edema can be severe.

Macroscopic Pathology

- The size varies from one to 20 cm. The average size is three centimeters.

Microscopic Pathology

- Skeletal muscles are observed with variable cell size.
- Dense fibrosis is common.
- Chronic inflammatory infiltration, especially the lymphocytes, is observed.
- Resitement of muscle with adipose tissue is observed in varying amounts.
- Atypia, calcification, or ossification are not observed.

Treatment

- Many cases are self-limiting and require treatment.

ELASTOFIBROMA

Definition

- Elastofibroma is a pseudo-degenerative tumor that is formed by overproduction of collagen and abnormal elastin fibers.

History

- First defined in 1961 by Jarvi & Saxen as elastofibroma. It was later renamed elastofibroma because it was also found in the affected areas.

Epidemiology

- Maximum prevalence: in the 6th and 7th decades.
- F> M.
- Most have a severe and long history.
- Elastofibroma-like cases are found in 13 to 17% of autopsies.

Clinical Signs

- It is most often found in the connective tissue between the chest and the scapular infromedial angle.
- As a slow-growing deep mass that can, in rare cases, cause pain, tenderness, and limited scapular movement or snap.
- Located deep in the rhomboid major and latissimus dorsi.
- Attached to the periosteum and adjacent ligaments of ribs 6, 7, and 8.
- 10% is bilateral.

Imaging

Increasingly, radiologists are discovering on Ct or MRI as a lesion of indefinite extent, heterogeneity with a skeletal muscle-like signal containing a striated or tumor-like fat signal.

Macroscopic Pathology

- Indeterminate, stiff, spherical, or elliptical, about 5-10 cm.

- On the incision surface, small areas of fat tissue are observed between the gray fibrous and gray areas, which sometimes contain cystic changes.
- It may be mistaken by sarcoma due to indeterminate margin and infiltration of skeletal and periosteal muscles.

Microscopic Pathology

- An interwoven mixture of swollen collagen, eosinophils and elastin fibers in equal amounts.
- There is also a small number of fibroblasts and fat cells of varying size.
- The elastic fibers have a degenerative, glossy appearance or are rarely fragmented into small flowers (Figure 5-27).
- Gomori and Verhoeff staining show fibers with and without branches that have a dense central core and an irregular willow fringe.

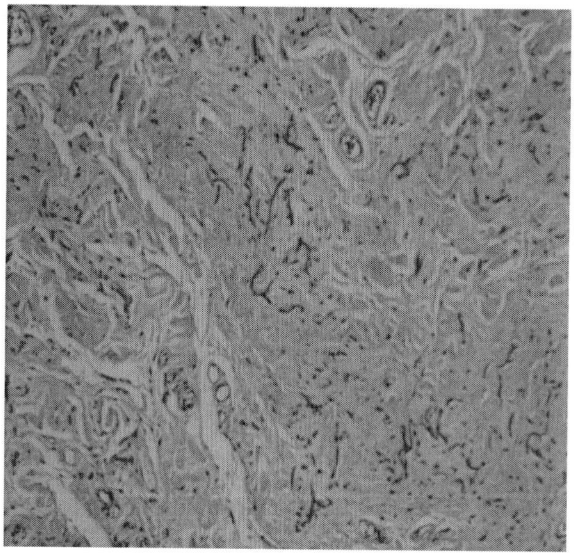

Figure 5-22.Elastofibroma: Collagen bundles alternate with large, thick eosinophilic elastic cylinders.

IHC

- Spindle-shaped cells are positive for vimentin.
- Actin, Desmin and S 100 are negative.

Differential Diagnosis

- Elastofibrolipoma: It has a definite margin, is surrounded by fibro capsules, has more adipose tissue in the central and peripheral parts.

Other

- Friction between the chest and the lower margin of the scapula can be effective.
- Some believe that cells of Periosteal origin produce elastofibroma in response to physical friction trauma.

- Most believe that fibroblasts and myofibroblasts are the source of abnormal elastic fibers.

Treatment

- Conservative removal of the tumor is an appropriate treatment. Recurrence is rare.
- Becoming malignant has not been reported.
- Can be diagnosed with the help of FNA or CNB.

Intramuscular Myxoma

- It is rare.
- Observed in adulthood.

It is usually found in the large muscles of the limbs.

- The tumor is common inside the heart and inside the heart is more common in the left vestibule.
- 5-10 cm at the time of diagnosis.
- Multiple form is less common and can be observed with multiple fibrous dysplasia, both of which occur in one area of the body (Mazabrad syndrome). This condition is more common on the right side of the body
- In Mazabrad syndrome, fibrous dysplasia is first diagnosed in adolescence and after 20 to 30 years, multiple myxomas appear.

MRI shows a low signal at T1 and a high signal at T2.

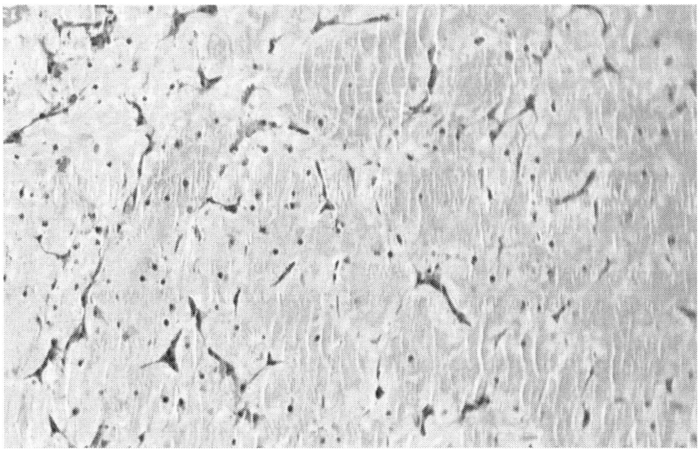

Figure 5-23. Myxoma: Stellate cells in an abundant myxoid matrix.

Chapter 6

Malignant Tumors of Soft Tissue

Undifferentiated Pleomorphic Sarcoma

Previous Name

- MFH

Epidemiology

- M = 2F
- Late adult age
- Most cases are observed between the ages of 50 and 70.
- It is more common in whites than in blacks.

Clinical Signs

- This diagnosis has to always be considered under the age of 20.
- Prevalence is more common in the thigh, upper limb, and posterior peritoneum.
- The inflammatory type is most often observed behind the peritoneum.
- Most often occurs as a growing painless mass.
- At the beginning of the diagnosis, most tumors are painless and larger than 5 cm.
- It has usually been involved the patient months and sometimes years before diagnosis.
- Tumor growth may increase suddenly.
- Like other sarcomas, growth spurts have been reported during pregnancy.
- There are constitutional signs in the posterior peritoneal type in contrast with the limb type: anorexia, weight loss, malaise, and increased abdominal pressure.
- Sometimes fever and leukocytosis with eosinophilia or neutrophilia are the predominant clinical features. This condition is especially observed in the inflammatory type of MFH and is caused by the production of cytotoxins such as IL-6, IL-8, and TNF. The above symptoms return due to tumor removal.

- Hypoglycemia is sometimes caused by ILGF-11.
- Metastasis may be observed at the same time with the primary tumor, but metastasis before the primary tumor are rare.

Etiology

- Like Atypical fibroxanthoma (which will be discussed later), many of these conditions are caused by radiotherapy and may occur years later.
- Bone insertion type of MFH has been observed following bone infarction or shrapnel bullets, or secondary to joint arthroplasties.

Imaging

- Cortical erosion due to a tumor, adjacent to the bone may be observed on the radiograph.
- MRI shows a marked mass or margin that is dark in T1 and bright in T2 (Figure 6-1).
- Large tumors of central necrosis are common on MRI.

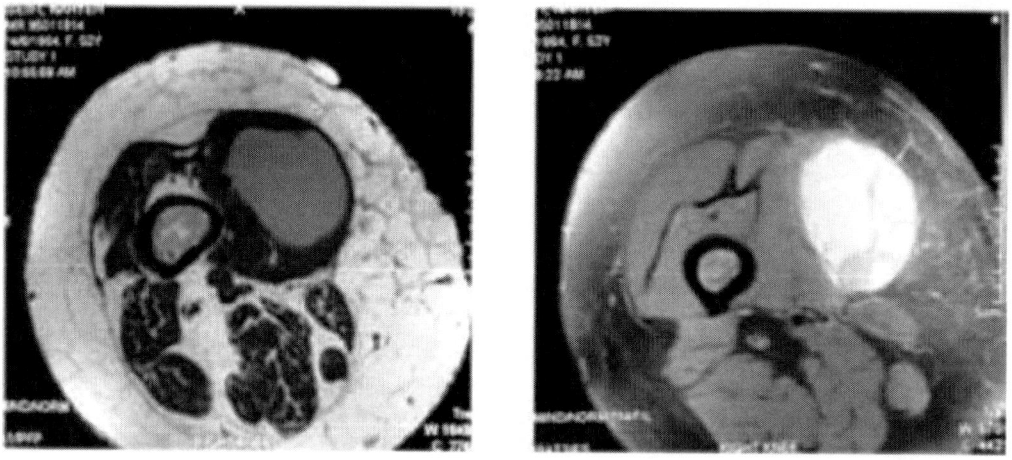

Figure 6-1. Left and right MRI T1 and T2, respectively, with fat suppressor from the MFH of the inferomedial thigh, where the heterogeneous lesion is observed as low signal and high signal, respectively.

Macroscopic Pathology

- Single lesion, multi-lobulated, flesh that is between 5 and 10 cm at the first time of diagnosis (Figure 6-2).
- Posterior peritoneal lesions are much larger than organ lesions at the time of diagnosis.
- 2.3 are found in skeletal muscle.
- Less than 10% are limited to subcutaneous.

- Despite macroscopically marginal, it can microscopically extend along fascial surfaces or between muscle fibers to a considerable distance from the primary tumor. Because of this, local recurrence is high.
- Gray to white on the surface cut.
- The inflammatory type has a yellow appearance due to the predominance of xanthoma cells, but hemorrhagic tumors are brown.
- The myxoid type is not macroscopically different from other myxoid tumors such as liposarcoma. Due to its mucoid appearance, it is translucent.
- Bleeding and necrosis are so common that 5% of these tumors are diagnosed as cystic hematomas due to extensive bleeding. Tumor cells are observed in the walls of these cysts.

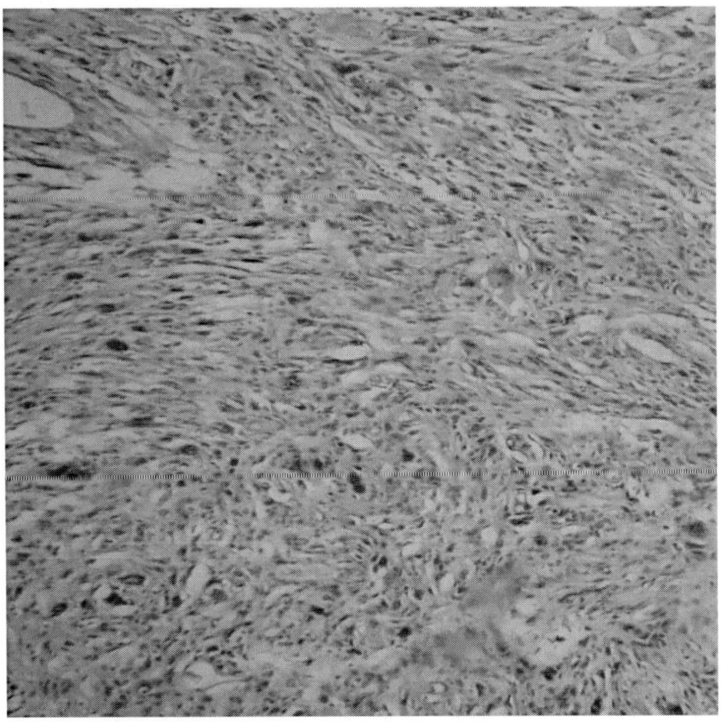

Figure 6-2. MFH: The characteristic feature of this tumor is the tornado appearance of spindle-shaped cells.

Microscopic Pathology

- It can be divided into 2 groups, Giant cell Storiform pleomorphic and inflammatory, but biological behavior is more related to tumor grade.
- Its pattern varies from storiform to pleomorphic.
- The stroma is made up of delicate collagen fibrils that surround individual cells.

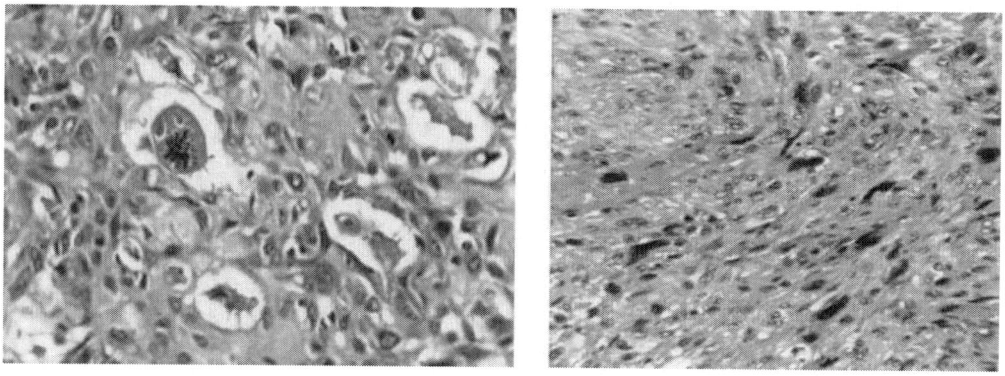

Figure 6-3. High magnification MFH: Represents mitosis and the pleomorphic nuclei.

Differential Diagnosis

- Pleomorphic liposarcoma: The presence of pleomorphic liposomes is characteristic.
- Liposarcoma without differentiation: It also has areas with good differentiation, which is characteristic. MFH is reported in the posterior peritoneal region of the liposarcoma without distinction in many cases, especially when the sample is insufficient.
- Pleomorphic leiomyosarcoma: It is very difficult to distinguish from MFH. Areas with smooth muscle differentiation help in diagnosis. The presence of an immune response to actin or, alternatively, amounts of actin and desmin in leiomyosarcoma is essential for diagnosis. In leiomyosarcoma, actin reactivity is common, but in MFH it is present only in peripheral areas due to the presence of myofibroblasts.
- Pleomorphic rhabdomyosarcoma: Severe cytoplasmic eosinophilia, cell-to-cell molding and the presence of strap cells are helpful.
- Anaplastic carcinoma: Especially important for posterior peritoneal lesions. It is also important for lesions in or near epithelial organs or lesions that occur in patients with a previous history of carcinoma.
- IHC staining is extremely important for pancytokeratin, which is positive in carcinoma and negative in MFH. However, keratin is found in a small percentage of MFH cases.

Other

- Local recurrence up to 30%.
- Metastasis up to 50%.
- 5-year survival 70-65%. In some studies, 5-year survival is reported to be less than 50%.
- Both local recurrence and metastasis occur in the first 12 to 24 months.

Common Sites of Metastasis Are

- Lung 90%
- Bone 8%
- Liver 1%

Bad Prognosis

- high depth

- large size
- High grade
- Metastasis
- Non-myxoid subtype
- Local recurrent necrosis

Myxoid Type

Definition

- Contains myxoid areas and cellular areas. Cell regions are not differentiable from normal MFH.

Differential Diagnosis

- The most important way to differentiate this tumor is to differentiate it from benign myxoid tumors such as nodular fasciitis and myxoma.
- Nodular fasciitis: May have focal myxoid changes but without a broad, regular vascular pattern, strangely shaped cells, and atrial fibrillation.
- Myxoma: It does not have the extensive MFH vascular pattern and cellular atypia and mitosis is so rare.
- Liposarcoma: Macroscopically, liposarcoma myxoid and MFH myxoid are similar, but myxoid liposarcoma consists of a homogeneous population of small spindle-shaped cells within a clear matrix. Liposarcoma does not have strangely shaped cells. Mitotic forms are uncommon and lipoblasts are common.
- Pleomorphic liposarcoma: Contains cells with strange shapes similar to MFH myxoid. But unlike MFH, the myxoid has a cellular background, not a myxoid, it contains lipoblasts, and the cells have a more homogeneous appearance.

Other

- Myxoid prognosis is better than storiform pleomorphic type.
- In order for this tumor to be called MFH myxoid, it has to have the following two characteristics:
- Have at least 50% of myxoid background tumors.
- Contains cells that resemble normal MFH.
- Recurrence is observed in 66% of the cases.
- Metastasis occurs in 25% of the cases.
- The time from diagnosis to metastasis in this type is longer.
- It is shallower and smaller than conventional MFH types.
- Being myxoid itself is good for prognosis.

Inflammatory MFH

- Observed entirely behind the peritoneum.
- Has prominent xanthomatous neutrophil infiltration. The latter causes the yellow appearance of the tumor.

Microscopic Pathology

- Xanthoma cells appear with a benign and malignant appearance, which is gigantic in size and the nucleus is strangely shaped.
- Neoplastic cells phagocytose neutrophils, unlike anaplastic lymphoma in which inflammatory cells do not phagocytose.

Differential Diagnosis

- Xanthogranulomatous pyelonephritis: Involves the kidneys early and most often and has symptoms of urinary tract infection. Culture in this tumor is necessary because infectious lesions are involved in its differential diagnosis. Atypia and mitotic activity are also observed in fibroblasts (in tumors).
- Lymphoma: Fever and leukemoid reaction are rare in lymphoma but may occur in inflammatory MFH. The IHC helps with the diagnosis. 50% local recurrence and 33% metastasis are observed in patients.

MFH Treatment

- Extensive resection is the treatment for this tumor.
- Radiotherapy is used in large tumors or when the resection margin is close to the tumor. It can be done before or after the operation. Preoperative radiotherapy is used for tumors that appear irreducible.
- Chemotherapy is used in most centers for large, high-grade soft tissue sarcomas, although its benefits have not been well established. In case of lung metastasis, chemotherapy is required in all soft tissue sarcomas.

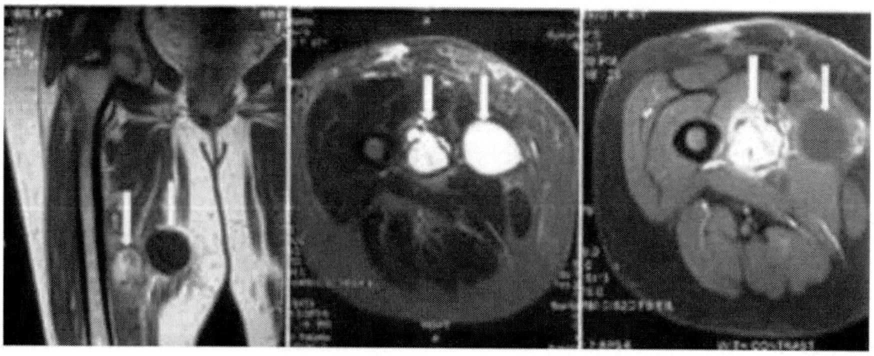

Figure 6-4. MRI of recurrence of MFH thigh in a 47-year-old woman. From left to right are T1, T2 with fat suppressor, and T1 with fat suppressor and contrast, respectively. In all three views, the left arrow indicates a recurrence of the tumor, and the right arrow indicates the accumulation of serous fluid at the site of previous surgery. Tumor recurrence has a nodular appearance and signal enhancement is observed using contrast, but seroma does not change signal (right figure) and is only limited to the seroma environment as the signal increases.

Liposarcoma

Definition

- A malignant adipose tissue tumor.

General Points

- The second common soft tissue sarcoma. In terms of prevalence, it constitutes 20% of soft tissue sarcomas.
- Most patients are over 50 years old.
- In no other group of sarcomas as much as liposarcoma does the pathologist see the necessity to divide liposarcoma into its subgroups.
- Liposarcomas are mostly located deep in the soft tissue, unlike lipomas, which are often found in superficial soft tissue.
- Liposarcomas are rarely observed in children. In children, there is lipoblastoma, which is a fetal type of lipoma.
- Liposarcoma is less likely to be caused by radiation.
- 49% in the organs. 41% in the lower extremities.
- 36% is behind the peritoneum.

Clinical Signs

- Large mass without deep pain in the limbs.
- Well Differentiated Type (WDL).

Another Name

- Atypical Lipomatosis Tumor. This name is given to limb tumors. The term well-differentiated liposarcoma is more appropriate behind the peritoneum and trunk.

Epidemiology

- Decades 6 and 7 have a maximum incidence.
- M = F.
- It is more common in men than women in the groin area.

Clinical Signs

- Painless deep mass with slow growth: occurs in the limbs. It existed months to years before the diagnosis. It is present in the proximal limb.
- Intra-abdominal mass: It occurs in those behind the peritoneum.
- Tends to local recurrence, but does not metastasize.
- It is considered malignant due to its high tendency for local recurrence.

Imaging

- Up to 75% of the tumor volume has a fat signal, similar to lipoma.
- They have more blurred margins than lipomas.
- There are thick septa or nodules inside them whose signal is the opposite of the fat signal. These areas become enhanced after the injection of the gadolinium contrast agent.

Macroscopic Pathology

- Large, multi-lumbar lesion varies from yellow to ivory.
- The difference with lipoma is in the following:
  - Much larger tumor size.
  - Existence of fibrous bands, gelatinous areas or bleeding points inside the tumor.

Microscopic Pathology

- Adipocytes of different sizes with fibrous septa.
- Cells have large hyperchromatic scattered nuclei.
- Stromal cells have an atypical appearance.

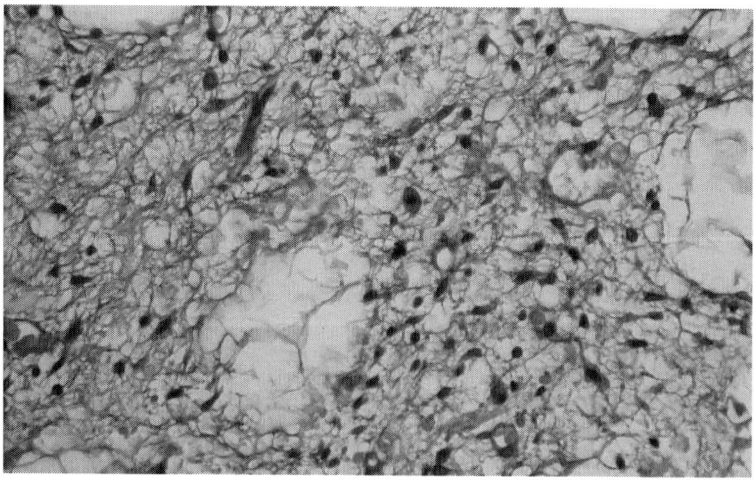

Figure 6-5. Atypical lipomatosis tumor: Adipocytes of different sizes with fibrous septa, Cells have large hyperchromatic scattered nuclei.

Differential Diagnosis

- Lipoma with fat necrosis: Macrophages are located near the degraded fat. Macrophages are also shaped and sized.
- Fat atrophy: Malnutrition, starvation, and localized trauma lead to fat atrophy.
- The cell shrinks and becomes epithelioid, the nuclei become more prominent, resembling lipoblasts.
- The differentiating point is that these fat cells have the same size, and this is unlike liposarcoma.
- Local massive lymphedema occurs in obese people due to chronic hanging of the fatty pannicalus.
- Symptoms of lymphedema include thickening of the superficial skin, fibrosis, edema, ectasia, and proliferation of lymph nodes and focal cysts.
- Reaction to silicon: Highly dilated multivacuum histyocitosis that mimic lipoblasts. It is observed in this case.
- The differential point is that in liposarcoma lipoblasts are not observed in such number and quality that these histosts are observed.
- Gravity free silicon can also be observed in areas far from the implantation area.
- Intramuscular lipoma with muscle atrophy.

Treatment and Clinical Behavior

- Treatment includes surgery alone.
- Patients are at risk for local recurrence, but metastasis is rare.
- The more inadequately the tumor is removed, the longer it stays and therefore the greater the chance of being dediffed: fewer superficial tumors than deep tumors and less deep ones than retroperitoneum.

DEDIFFERENTIATED LIPOSARCOMA

Epidemiology

- Their age group is similar to WDL.
- M = F.

Site

- Retroperitostum = 3 times more than the organs.

Imaging

- On Ct and MRI, they are observed as mass-like areas of non-adipose tissue, similar to other sarcomas, inside a fat-containing tumor.

Macroscopic Pathology

- It is observed as a large multinodular yellow mass (area with good differentiation) mixed with dentinal areas (foci of dedifferentiation).
- The margin between the two WDL regions and the Dedifferentiation region is quite sharp.

Microscopic Pathology

- Dedifferentiation zones in 90% of the cases are composed of fibrosarcoma or MFH.
- Leukemoid reaction has been reported in association with tumors containing MFH inflammatory foci.

Differential Diagnosis

- Sarcoma infltraing fat: It is difficult to differentiate between a pleomorphic sarcoma that infiltrates fat and a dediff liposarcoma.
- To diagnose dediff liposarcoma, there has to be foci of WDL somewhere in the tumor.
- The importance of differentiating between the two:
- Minimal dedifferentiation for the term dedifferentiation, it has to be macroscopically more than one centimeter from the tumor.

Clinical Behavior

- Slightly better than other high-grade sarcomas in adults.
- 41% have a local recurrence, 17% have metastasis, and 28% die from the tumor within five years.
- Most patients die from the local complications of their tumor before the onset of distant metastasis.
- The site of the tumor is the most important prognostic factor, which has the worst prognosis in the posterior peritoneal region.
- In posterior peritoneal tumors, rhabdomyoblast differentiation is associated with a very short lifespan.

Liposarcoma Myxoid

- It is 1.2 to 1.3% of all liposarcomas (45 to 55%).
- The peak age is in the fifth decade (average age 42 years).
- It is 75% in the lower extremities, especially the medial thigh and pelvis.
- They tend to occur behind the peritoneum, so a CT scan of the chest, abdomen, and pelvis is recommended for staging and follow-up of patients.
- It occurs with a painless mass with slow growth in the lower extremities.

Imaging

- Heterogeneously observed on CT. Nesfield numbers are higher than fat and less than muscle.

- MRI: The whole tumor is low signal due to high water content in T1, but the fat part is more than High signal. 90% of the tumor is composed of a base material that has high water content.
- Observed as a high signal in T2 view.

Macroscopic Pathology

- Multinodular gelatinous mass usually has no necrosis but sometimes contains hemorrhages

Microscopic Pathology

- The pure myxoid type is very similar to developing fetal fat.
- It is a low cellularity multinodular mass that is slightly more cellular in the periphery.
- Bleeding may be so severe that the tumor is mistaken with Hemangioma.
- Bone, cartilage, or smooth muscle differentiation may be observed and has no effect on prognosis.
- By losing differentiation, the cells take on a round cell appearance.
- 90% of the tumor is composed of ground substance.

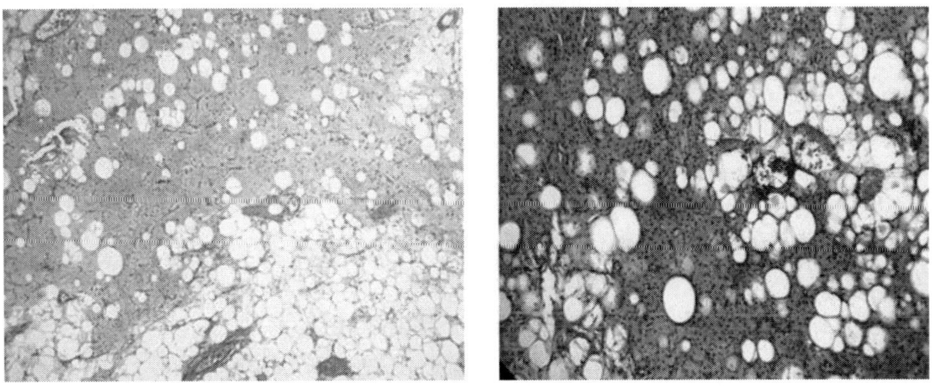

Figure 6-6. Myxoid liposarcoma: Cells are found in a network of finely branched capillaries.

Treatment and Clinical Behavior

- Wide resection treatment.
- Adjuvant radiotherapy has been reported to be helpful.
- Except for synovial sarcoma, it is the only adult soft tissue sarcoma in which chemotherapy is useful.
- 5-year survival is 90-80% in low-grade types.
- Tends to metastasize to other areas of the body that contain fat (mediastinum, pelvic bone marrow, and spine).
- For the above reasons, patients has to be staged and followed up by CT scan of the chest, abdomen and pelvis.

Pleomorphic Liposarcoma

- Less than 5% of liposarcomas. It is the rarest subgroup of liposarcoma.
- Very malignant.

- Always have a lot of mitoses.
- Observed in the elderly.
- The most common site is the deep tissue of the limbs.
- Premature metastasis is common and almost always metastasizes to the lungs.
- The use of chemotherapy has to be discussed with the patient on a case-by-case basis.

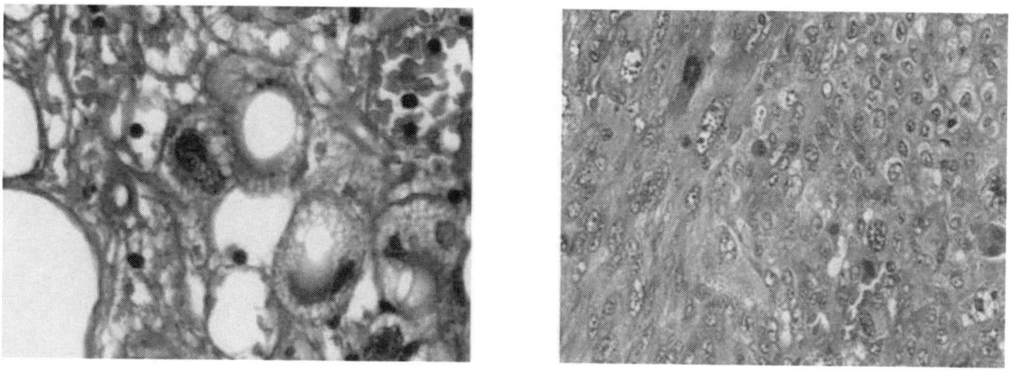

Figure 6-7. Pleomorphic liposarcoma: The nuclei of the cells of this tumor are larger, more colorful, and more diverse than normal lipoblasts.

- Poor prognosis in liposarcomas
- High grade
- Large size
- Depth site
- Existence of metastasis

Synovial Sarcoma

Definition

- Malignant neoplasm of spindle-shaped mesenchymal cells with variable epithelial differentiation involving gland formation. This tumor is characterized by chromosomal transit t (X; 18) (p11; q11).

General Points

- It is very rare in the joints and is found mainly in the para-articular areas of the limbs, especially in the immediate vicinity of the tendon sheet, bursae, and joint capsule. Less than 10% of the cases are observed in the joint or in relation to the joint.

Types

- Type B phase 1: They have epithelial and spindle cell components. With variable ratios.
- Monophase type 1: It covers about two thirds of the cases.
- Poorly differentiated type: which may be confused with Ewing's sarcoma or rhabdomyosarcoma.

Epidemiology

- It is mainly observed in the age group of 15 to 40 years.
- The average age is 34 years.
- 44% are less than 30 years old at the time of diagnosis.
- M ÷ F = 1.2.

Clinical Signs

- Tactile deep mass with pain or tenderness.
- At the beginning of diagnosis, the size of this tumor is less than 5 cm.
- Less commonly, pain or tenderness are the only symptoms of the disease.
- A slight decrease in the range of motion of the adjacent joint may be observed.
- Weight loss is rare. If present, it is associated with large, long-term, and poorly differentiated masses.
- Paresthesia and nerve pain due to nerve involvement may exist.
- The duration of symptoms in most cases is 2 to 4 years.
- Rarely, there have been cases for up to 20 years before surgery.

Relationship with Trauma and Environmental Factors

- The interval between the history of trauma and the onset of the disease was a few weeks to 40 years. The association with trauma is incidental. Synovial sarcoma is more common in areas prone to trauma.
- Rarely observed in the radiotherapy field.
- It is one of the tumors, associated with meta implant in THA.

Anatomical Site

- Mostly in the limbs. They are located near the large joints in the limbs, especially the knees.

- It is very rare in the joints and is found mainly in the paraarticular areas of the limbs, especially in the immediate vicinity of tendon sheets, bursae and joint capsules. The tumor is usually attached to tendons, joint capsules, or tendon sheets.
- In less than 10% of the cases, it is observed in the joint or in relation to the joint. Intra-articular type: covers less than 5% of the cases.
- It is more common in the lower extremities than the upper extremities. It is mostly around the knee. The most common soft tissue sarcoma in the foot.
- 15% is observed in the upper limb in the same proportion around its joints.
- 5 to 10% is found in the head and neck. After the limbs, it is the most common site of conflict.
- 5% is found in the trunk.
- Synovial sarcoma has been reported anywhere in the body, even inside the heart.

Imaging

- Swelling of oval or spherical tissue may be observed on plain radiograph (Figure 6-13).
- 15 to 20% of periosteal reactions, superficial bone erosion or bone invasion are observed.
- Extensive bone destruction is observed in long-term large or poor diff types.
- 15 to 20% focal calcification, mostly fine stippling. Sometimes large areas of the tumor are radiopaque.
- Radiopaque appearance is not observed in other soft tissue sarcomas, except in extra-skeletal osteosarcoma and synovial sarcoma.
- MRI is dark on T1 and bright on T2.

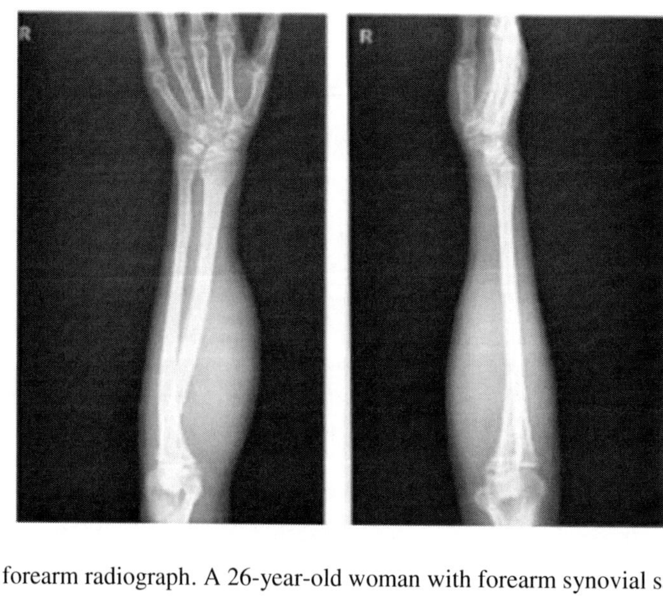

Figure 6-8. Plain forearm radiograph. A 26-year-old woman with forearm synovial sarcoma.

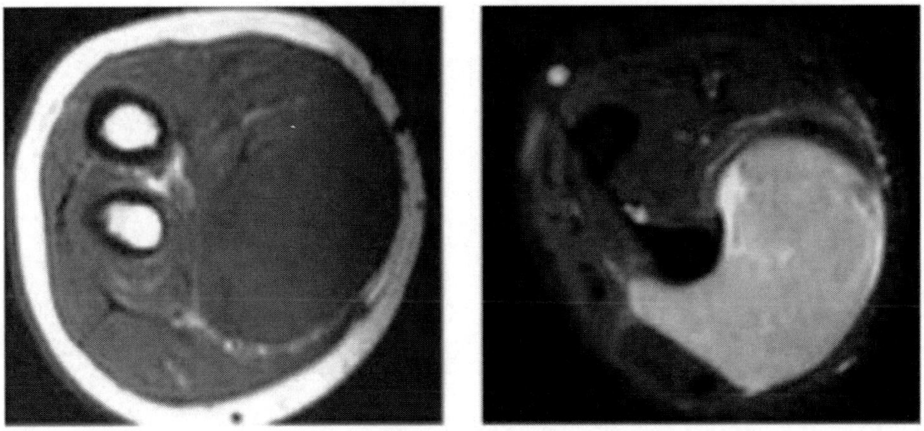

Figure 6-9. Patient forearm MRI from left to right T1 and T2 with fat suppressor that the lesion is Low signal and High signal, respectively.

Macroscopic Pathology

- False capsules are most often observed in slow-growing lesions, which are often shiny.
- The formation of cysts inside the tumor may be obvious and sometimes occurs as multicysts (Figure 6-15).
- Depending on the collagen content, they are soft or hard to the touch.
- They are yellow to white-gray on the cutting surface.
- They are usually three to six centimeters at the time of excision (although up to 15 centimeters has been observed).
- Less differentiated type: observed fragile with multiple cystic areas or bleeding and necrosis. Hemorrhagic types may be confused with organized hematoma or angiosarcoma.

Microscopic Pathology

- Unlike most other sarcomas, this tumor is made up of two different types of cells: epithelial cells that look like carcinoma cells and spindle-shaped cells.
- The monophasic type of tumor involves the monotone proliferation of spindle-shaped cells arranged in long, nested fascicles. Nuclear pleomorphicism or necrosis is not commonly observed.
- 97% positive for cytokeratin.

Types

- Biophysics: which have varying amounts of both cell types. The classic type is synovial sarcoma. It covers a third of the cases.
- Monophasic: accounts for about two-thirds of the cases. In terms of prognosis, there is no difference between the two types.

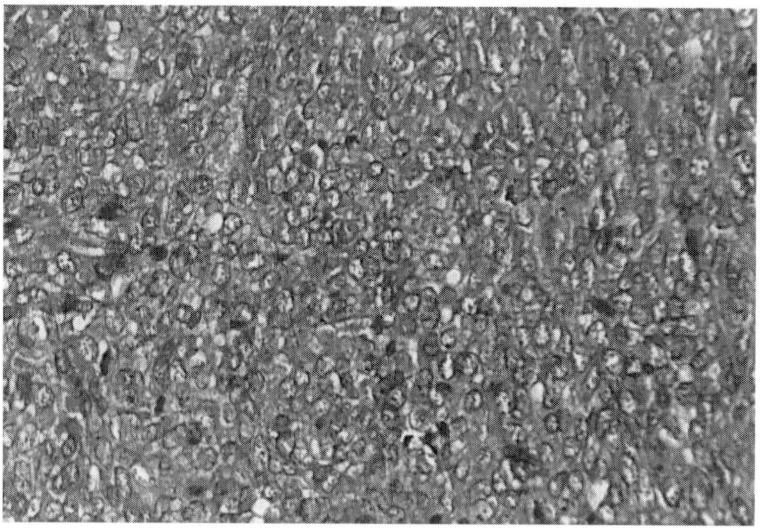

Figure 6-10. Synovial sarcoma: Islets of epithelioid cells.

Metastasis and Recurrence

- 80% recurrence is observed in surgery with insufficient margin and without adjuvant treatment.
- Recurrence of less than 40% has been observed in surgery with sufficient margin or with adjuvant radiotherapy.
- Recurrence is mainly in the first 2 years.
- Metastasis of about 50% to:
- Lung → Lymph nodes → Bone marrow.
- Lymph node metastasis is observed in 20% of the cases. It is recommended to pay attention to the lymph nodes during the physical examination.

Table 6-1. Risk of metastasis

	Low	**High**
Age	< 25	> 40
size	$< 5\ cm$	$\leq 5\ cm$
Poorly diff	$-$	$+$
Area	Distal	Proximal

Treatment

- Sensitive to chemotherapy.
- Treatment includes wide excision and adjuvant therapy.
- Radiotherapy is recommended for large tumors that are initially considered inoperable before surgery. Radiotherapy is recommended for tumors larger than five centimeters, before or after surgery.
- Chemotherapy is recommended for metastatic patients or tumors larger than five centimeters after surgery.

Differential Diagnosis

- Malignant peripheral nerve sheath tumor.
- Dermatofbrosarcoma protuberans.

Bad Prognosis

- Size larger than five centimeters.
- Age over 40 years.
- Differentiation.

Good Prognosis

- Distal lesions have a better clinical outcome than proximal.
- The highly calcified type generally has a better long-term outcome.

EPITHELOID SARCOMA

Definition

- Malignant neoplasm of soft tissue with slow growth and aggression. This tumor involves the superficial soft tissue, tendons, and tendon sheets and has a firm consistency.

Epidemiology

- Occurs in adolescents and young adults.
- The average age of the conflict is 26 to 29 years.
- It twice more common in men than in women.

Common Site

- It is more common in distal limbs, especially upper limbs and hands and fingers.
- The most common soft tissue sarcoma is the hand.

Clinical Signs

- Most often observed on flexor surfaces of fingers, hands and forearms.
- In the form of one or more nodules without pain and hard surface with woody consistency.
- Its average size is three centimeters.
- Superficial nodules commonly cause skin lesions and are mistakenly treated as infected warts.

Imaging

- MRI can be a mass with a definite or indeterminate margin. It commonly affects the skin and superficial soft tissue.
- Low / intermediate: T1 signal.
- Intermediate / high: T2 signal.
- May be solid or have one or more fluid levels.
- Solid tumor areas with gadolinium increase absorption.

Macroscopic Pathology

- Tumor size varies from 0.5 to 5 cm.
- Deep tumors are usually larger and do not appear as rigid multinodular masses with irregular margins.
- The cutting surface is gray-white or gray-bronze and shiny.
- Yellow or brown focal areas are observed due to bleeding or necrosis.

Microscopic Pathology

- Tumor cells are nodularly arranged.
- They tend to degenerate or have central necrosis.
- They have an epithelial appearance in which the cytoplasm of cells is eosinophilic.
- The nodular appearance is more pronounced in specimens taken from tumor recurrence.
- Necrosis of tumor nodules, which is more pronounced in the center, is a common finding.
- Tumors can grow along neurovascular bundles.
- Extensive tumors that spread to the dermis or those that have been in the dermis for the first time often injure the skin and form SCC (squamous cell carcinoma).
- There are two general types of cells: epithelioid cells and spindle-shaped cells. It has to be noted that the pattern does not exist with the physical phase of the cells and the two types of cells are mixed with each other and are not observed separately, so avoid synovial sarcoma.

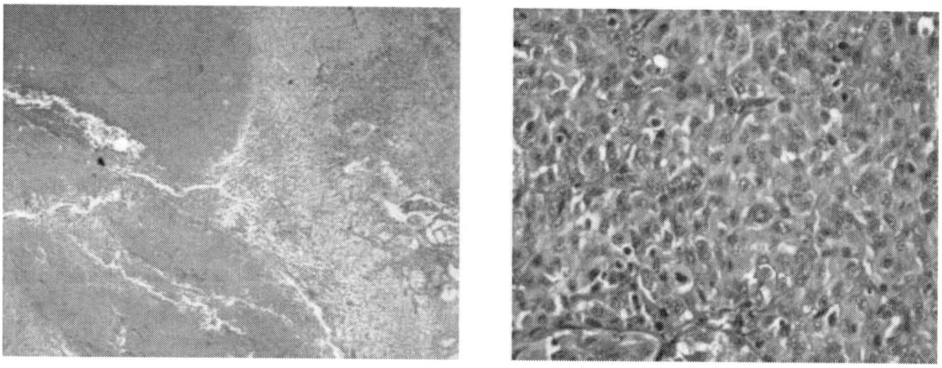

Figure 6-11. Epithelioid sarcoma: Left side: Central necrosis, Right side: The epithelial cells are clustered with eosinophilic cytoplasm and large cells.

Treatment

- Includes resection or amputation with wide margin.
- Chemotherapy is used only for metastatic disease.
- Local recurrence and metastasis are high and both may be observed for years after initial diagnosis.
- After the lungs, the most common sites are lymph node metastasis. It is recommended to pay attention to the lymph nodes during the physical examination.

Bad prognostic factors include:

- Male sex.
- Larger size or equal to 5 cm.
- Proximal site in the limbs.
- More tumor depth.
- Bleeding inside the tumor.
- Necrosis inside the tumor.
- High mitotic index.
- Invasion of blood vessels.
- Inadequate primary excision.

Differential Diagnosis

- An inflammatory process such as rheumatoid nodule or nodular fasciitis: Separated cells in the sarcoma epithelium have more specific margins, larger, and more eosinophilic.
- Malignant schwannoma: S100 staining is positive and cytokeratin staining is negative, both of which are in contrast to the condition observed in sarcoma epithelium.
- Malignant melanoma: S100 and Melan A staining is positive in melanoma, which is negative in sarcoma epithelium.
- Injured SCC: The sarcoma epithelium, unlike scc, does not have keratin pearl and dyskeratosis in the adjacent epithelium. It is negative for CD5/6 but SCC is positive.

Dermatofibrosarcoma Protobrans

Definition

- A malignant neoplasm is a nodular soft tissue that appears just below the epidermis in the form of one or more nodules and may grow into a large mass.

Epidemiology

- It is observed in young or middle-aged adults.
- M> F.

- Due to the slow growth of the tumor, it may have been present in some cases from childhood and has manifested in young adults.

Common Site

- It is more common in the trunk and proximal organs (unlike epithelioids sarcoma).

Clinical Signs

- It has a slow and continuous growth for many years.
- In the early stages: The plaque-like mass appears on the skin with a red or blue discoloration of the upper skin.
- In the final stages, with increasing tumor growth, a prominent appearance is observed.
- The skin on the tumor is easily injured.

Macroscopic Pathology

- Gray-white lumps are prominent on the skin and subcutaneous tissue.
- The average size during surgery is usually 5 cm.
- Multiple lumps or nodules are more common in recurrent lesions.
- The skin on the tumor is stretched or injured.
- Expansion to the striated muscles is rare with the exception of large or recurrent tumors.
- Gelatinous areas inside the tumor that are caused by myxoid changes are sometimes observed.
- Bleeding and cystic changes are sometimes observed inside the tumor.

Microscopic Pathology

- The tumor diffusely infiltrates the skin and subcutaneous tissue.
- Slender, fibroblast cells that have accumulated in a whirlwind (clearly storiform view) around the arteries are a hallmark of this tumor.
- Nuclear pleomorphism and mitosis are rare.
- Secondary elements such as Xanthoma cell, Giant cell and inflammatory components are rare.
- In the presence of myxoid changes, accumulations of the underlying substance are found between the cells.
- Mitotic activity in dermatofibrosarcoma is less than 5 mitoses per HPF (high power field) but higher in fibrosarcoma.

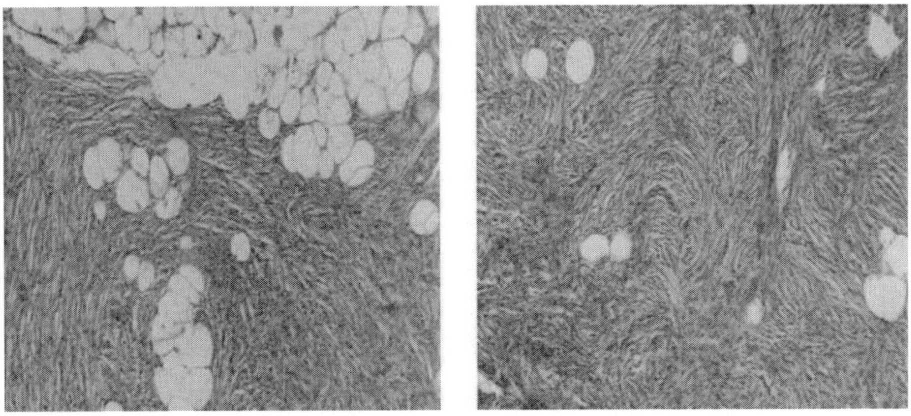

Figure 6-12. Dermatofibrosarcoma protuberans: with subcutaneous fat infiltration.

Treatment

Treatment includes wide resection. With skin defect reconstruction (in areas where the surrounding soft tissue is insufficient to cover the defect, such as the back of the feet and hands).

- Recurrence occurs in up to 50% of the cases and the reason for the high recurrence is extensive infiltration of the skin by the tumor which may not be noticed during surgery and may result in insufficient margin.
- With wide excision, recurrence occurs in 10 to 20%. More precisely:
  - If the margin is greater or equal to 3 cm, the recurrence is about 20% and if the margin is less or equal to 2 cm, the recurrence is about 42%.
- Despite being locally aggressive, this tumor rarely metastasizes.

Tumors of Striated Muscle Origin

Rhabdomyosarcoma

Definition

- Primarily occurs in soft tissue. Very rarely observed in bone.

Types of:

- Embryonic: 50 to 70%.
- Alveolar: 18 to 45%.
- Pleomorphic: 5 to 10%.
- Embryonic and alveolar are mainly observed in children and pleomorphic are observed mainly in adults.

Epidemiology

- Age: Observed between 2 and 40 years old with an average age of 18 years.
- Slightly more common in males.
- The most common sarcoma is pediatric soft tissue.

Site

- Alveolar and pleomorphic: More common in organs.
- Embryonic: The cervix is involved in 74% of the cases.

Clinical Signs

- Embryonic: A soft, rapidly growing tissue mass that manifests itself as signs of compaction of adjacent structures. Proptosis, diplopia, sinusitis are the symptoms.
- Alveolar: A soft tissue mass with rapid growth in the head and neck or limbs. Like the previous type, it is associated with squeezing adjacent buildings. Lymph node metastasis is more common in this type than in other types of rhabdomyosarcoma.
- Pleomorph: A soft tissue mass with rapid growth in the organs. It is painful too.

Macroscopic Pathology

- Embryonic: Earphone in tan color with unspecified margin. The botryoid type has a polypoid appearance and is observed with clusters of nodules near the surface of the epithelium.
- Alveolar: fleshy and fibrous, gray-white or gray-tan.
- Pleomorphic: White-gray with varying degrees of necrosis and bleeding. These tumors are large (5 to 15 cm) and often have fibrous pseudocapsules. Their margins can be definite or indefinite.

Microscopic Pathology

- Embryonic: bundles of spindle cells with hyperchromatic or vesicular bones and abundant eosinophilic cytoplasm. In most cases the spindle cell component is prominent. It is composed of high-cell and low-cell regions. Cellular regions are located in the form of cell clusters around the arteries.

Imaging

- May have erosion or bone destruction (cortex / medulla).
- Calcification is uncommon.

CT Scan

- Have a definite or indeterminate margin.

MRI

- Ovoid or lobulated.
- Margin is clear or uncertain.
- T1: low signal
- T2: intermediate/high signal

Bone scan: Part of the diagnostic procedure before rhabdomyosarcoma treatment is because this tumor has the ability to metastasize to the bone, even in children.

Differential Diagnosis

- Liposarcoma
- Leiomyosarcoma

Treatment

- In all types: extensive resection or amputation with pre- and postoperative chemotherapy and radiotherapy.
- In the embryonic type, with metastasis in the initial diagnosis: they have a 5-year survival of 20 percent. Absence of metastasis: 64 to 95% have a 5-year survival.
- •Alveolar: 53% have 5-year survival.

Pleomorph: 70% of patients die within 20 months. Poor prognosis.

LEIOMYOSARCOMA

Definition

- A malignant mesodermal tumor is differentiated into smooth muscle.

Epidemiology

- The most common age of conflict is 35 to 79 years and an average of 58 years.
- The primary intraosseous type is about 10 years younger (middle age).
- M = F.
- Posterior peritoneal type is 1.5 times more common in women than men.
- It is generally rare.

Conflict Site

- In order of high to low prevalence: posterior peritoneum, lower limbs, hips and buttocks, trunk, upper limbs, feet and ankles, other areas.
- Bone type: Inside the femur, the distal part is the most common site of involvement.
- Its soft tissue type is much more common than its intraosseous type.

Clinical Signs

- Local swelling of soft tissue with or without pain for days to years.
- Pain is the most common symptom in the intraosseous type.

Imaging

- Observed as a soft tissue mass.
- Rarely contains mineralization.
- The intraosseous type is radiolucent with a permeative or moth-eaten appearance. Sometimes geographically. Periosteal reaction is rare.

MRI

- Margin can be definite or indefinite.
- T1: low/intermediate.
- T2: intermediate/high.
- Areas of necrosis or cystic change (in large tumors) are observed as low T1 signal and high T2 signal.
- Moderate/high enhancement is observed in the cellular areas of the tumor after Gadolinium injection.
- Bone lesions are similar to soft tissue lesions in terms of signal changes on MRI.

Macroscopic Pathology

- Tumor size varies, often being large.
- Posterior peritoneal tumors are often larger than 10 cm and limb tumors are smaller than 10 cm.
- On the cutting surface is gray tan.
- Bleeding and necrosis are common in tumors.
- It is often associated with and originates from large blood vessels.

Microscopic Pathology

- The tumor is composed of highly eosinophilic bundles or spindle cell clusters.
- The nucleus of cells, like smooth muscle cells, is long and has a rounded end that gives it the appearance of a cigarette.
- Has a lot of mitoses.
- Pleomorphism is a variable nucleus.

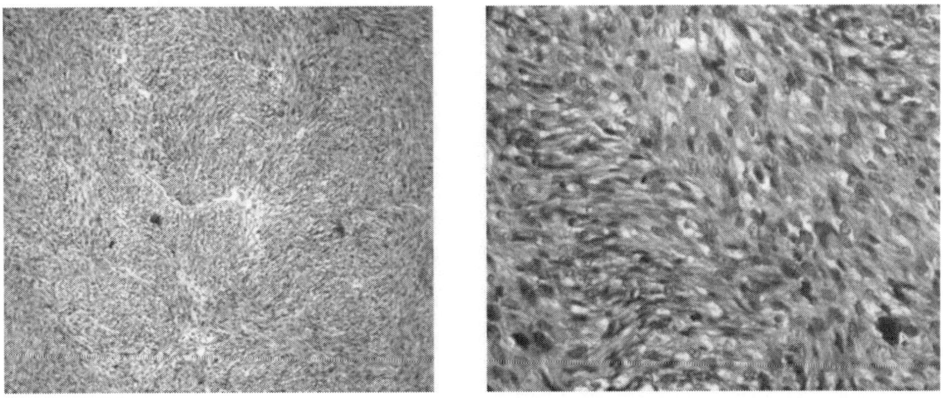

Figure 6-13. Leiomyosarcoma. Accumulations of spindle-shaped cells are Characteristic of this tumor. The cells are like smooth muscle cells, long and have a round end. The cytoplasm of the cells is strongly eosinophilic.

Differential Diagnosis

- Soft tissue type: MFH, synovial sarcoma, fibrosarcoma, indiscriminate liposarcoma, schwannoma, neurofibroma, rhabdomyosarcoma, desmoid tumor.
- Bone lesions: metastasis, myeloma, lymphoma, MFH, chondrosarcoma, osteosarcoma.

Treatment and Disease Course

- Treatment includes surgery with radiotherapy or chemotherapy.
- The posterior peritoneal type is larger than the peripheral types of the disease. It metastasizes more commonly and has a worse prognosis.
- The most common areas for metastasis are the lungs.
- 5-year survival for peripherals is 64%.
- 5-year survival is lower for the posterior peritoneal type.
- Prognosis is better in children than in adults because low-grade tumors are more common.

Other

- It can be primary or observed after radiotherapy.
- Malignant tumor of the peripheral nerve sheath.
- Malignant peripheral nerve sheath tumors (MPNSTs).

DEFINITION

Another Name Is Neurofibrosarcoma

- The current name is MPNSTs.

Epidemiology

- In non-neurofibromatosis cases, men and women are equally involved.
- In cases of neurofibromatosis, men are four times more likely to be involved than women.
- Most cases are observed in the range of 30 to 50 years. Thus: it is observed in patients with neurofibromatosis at a younger age and in those who do not have neurofibromatosis at an older age. In one study, the median age of patients was 33 years and was more common in the men.

Clinical Signs

- 25% to 50% of patients with this tumor have neurofibromatosis. The rest, which accounts for about two-thirds of the cases, are sporadic.
- 3 to 5% of people with neurofibromatosis develop MPNSTs, and if pain occurs in a previous neurofibroma, the doctor has to consider it as a transformation to MPNSTs.
- Other neurological tumors, including cutaneous neurofibromas, neurofibroma plexiform, and glioma optic are more common in neurofibromatosis.
- Most patients have an increasingly painful mass. Pain is more common in those with neurofibromatosis.
- In cases of neurofibromatosis, they appear about 10 to 20 years after diagnosis.
- About 10 to 20% of the cases occur after radiation exposure (therapeutic/occupational) and with a dormant period of about 15 years.

Site

- Most cases occur in large nerve trunks, including the sciatic nerve, brachial plexus, and sacral plexus. Therefore, proximal upper and lower limbs and trunk are the most common areas involved.

Note:

- The presence of pain or sudden enlargement of a mass that already exists in patients with neurofibromatosis necessitates an immediate biopsy, as MPNST is usually more painful in the setting of neurofibromatosis.

- Referral, mild, and paraesthetic pain may present as a combination of symptoms. This is where MPNST originates in the major nerve.

Macroscopic Pathology

- Large eccentric mass in a major nerve.
- Thickening of the nerve in the proximal and distal to the mass indicates the spread of the neoplasm along the epineurium and perineurium.
- Most cases of MPNST that occur in the setting of neurofibromatosis are caused by deep, not superficial, neurofibromas.
- The appearance of the tumor is similar to other soft tissue sarcomas. On the cutting surface of the flesh-white-opaque facade (not bright) with areas of bleeding and necrosis.

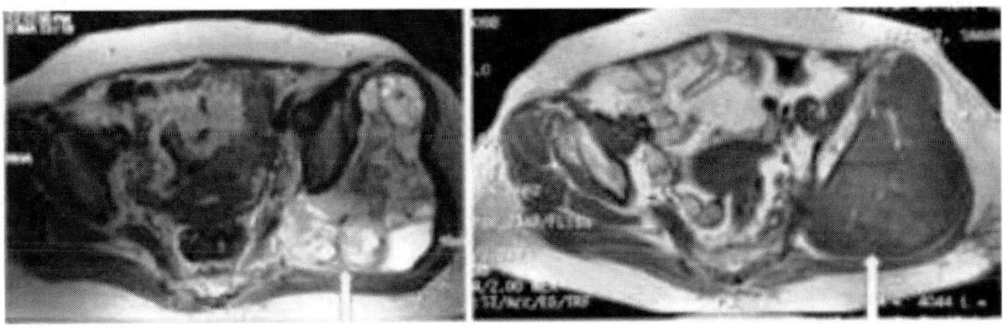

Figure 6-14. MPNST in the sciatic nerve in the sciatic notch (arrows). From left to right, MRI shows T1 and T2, where the tumor is heterogeneous high signal and low signal, respectively

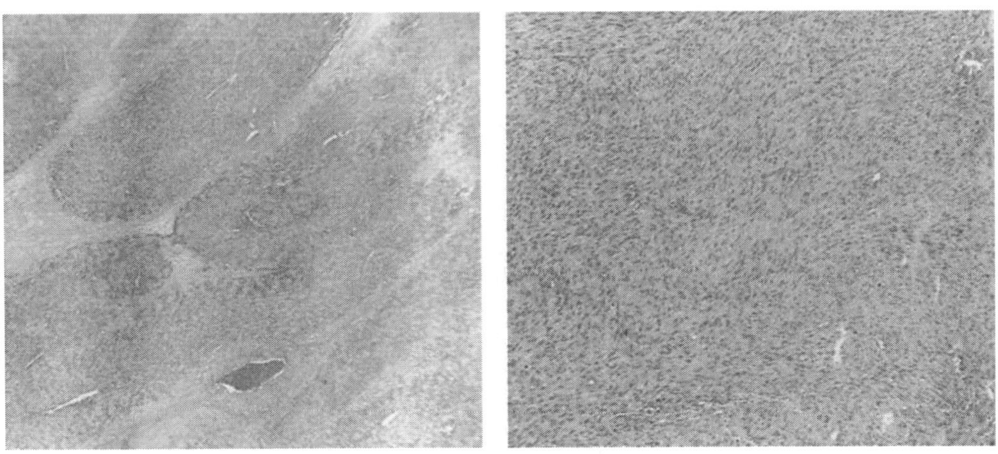

Figure 6-15. MPNST: The large areas of geographic necrosis that characterize this tumor. Intertwined fascicles of identical spindle cells with multicolored nuclei and abundant mitosis.

Microscopic Pathology

- The general appearance is similar to fibrosarcoma with specific changes.
- Tumor cells largely retain the Schwann appearance from which they are originated.

- The nuclei of cells in the longitudinal cut are wavy or comma-shaped. When transverse cut, they are elliptically asymmetrical.
- The cytoplasm is indistinct and has little staining.
- The cells are arranged in intertwined fascicles.
- Nuclear palisading can occur locally in less than 10% of all MPNSTs.
- Mitosis is common.
- The most common Heterogeneous elements are the mature islets of cartilage and bone. They are found in 10 to 15% of MPNST, and this rate is higher than all other types of sarcomas.

Treatment and Clinical Behavior

- The main treatment for this tumor is surgery and it has a high morbidity due to its origin from large nerves. In some cases, recurrence has been observed in healthy areas of the nerve after complete removal of the tumor. About one-third of patients require amputation initially or as a result of recurrence.

Bad prognosis is associated with:

- The size of the tumor is large.
- The tumor is not in the limb.
- High Grade/stage
- Necrosis is inside the tumor.
- Caused by radiation.
- The surgical margin is positive.
- If the above cases are the same, tumors that develop in patients with neurofibromatosis do not have a worse prognosis than those in patients without neurofibromatosis.
- In general, local recurrence and metastasis is about 40 to 65%.
- The overall 5-year survival is about 52%.
- The most common site of metastasis is the lungs, followed by the bones and pleura.

Metastasis is very common in this tumor.

- And is more common than other soft tissue sarcomas.
- Less than 10% of the cases metastasize to the local lymph nodes, so routine removal of the local lymph nodes during tumor surgery is not necessary. Radiotherapy is standard in large tumors (larger than five centimeters). Even with radiotherapy, the recurrence is high. Chemotherapy is used in cases of metastatic disease, although the response of this tumor to chemotherapy is low.

Other

- In animals, if ethylnitrosourea is injected transplacental, it can cause sarcoma.

EXTRAOSSEOUS OSTEOSARCOMA

Definition

- A malignant mesenchymal neoplasm that forms osteoid, bone or chondroid and is found in soft tissue without adhesion to the skeleton.

Epidemiology

- It is rare.
- It accounts for 1 to 2% of all osteosarcomas.
- Rarely observed under 40 years. The most common age is over 40 years.
- M ÷ F = 1.9.

Common Site

- The thigh muscles are the most common site of involvement.
- The muscles of the pelvic girdle and shoulder girdle and the posterior peritoneal region are the next most common.

Clinical Signs

- Large soft tissue masses are a common symptom.
- There is pain in 1/3 of the cases.
- Injuries are observed only in chronic and large tumors after the biopsy.
- Most patients present 6 to 8 months after the onset of symptoms.
- Cases of extraskeletal osteosarcoma following radiotherapy and most commonly for breast cancer has been observed. These tumors appear 4 years or more after primary tumor radiotherapy.

Imaging

- Soft tissue mass may be visible on the radiograph.
- Spotty or bulky calcification.
- No bone involvement.

Macroscopic Pathology

- Can have a definite margin with a false capsule.
- Can be infiltrative with indeterminate margins.

- On the surface white and granular with yellow spots with numerous foci of bleeding and necrosis is observed.
- Most tumors were 5 to 10 cm in size during surgery.

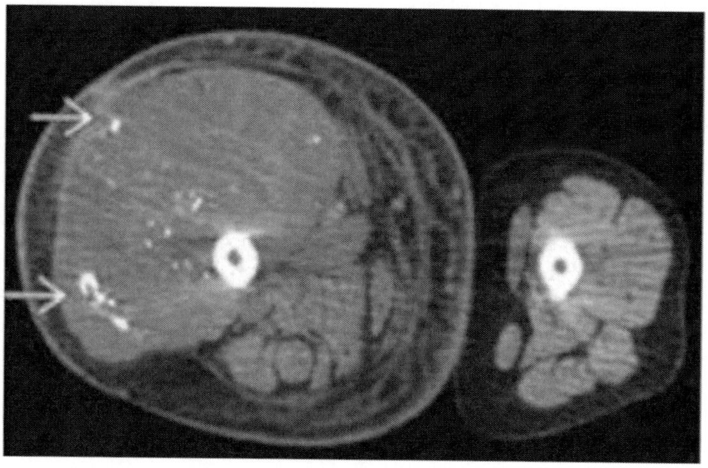

Figure 6-16. Osteosarcoma outside the bone. The tumor typically presents as a massive mass of soft tissue, usually in the thigh muscles, with calcifications (arrows) similar to those observed on this CT scan.

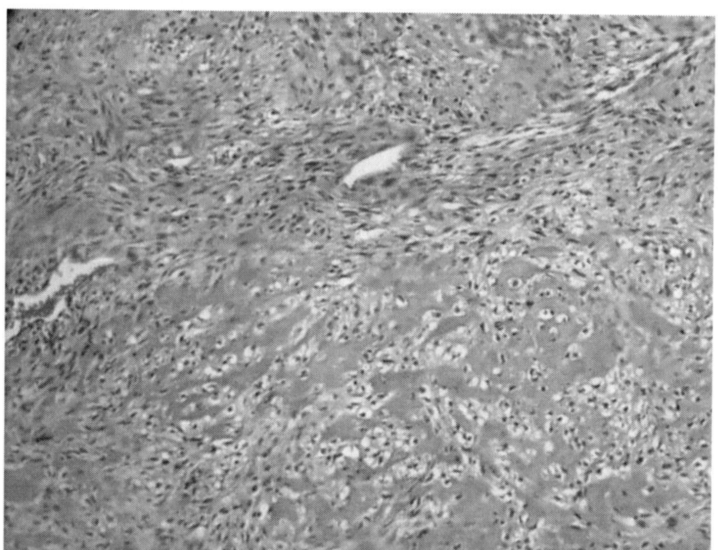

Figure 6-17. Extraosseous osteosarcoma: The net-like osteoid matrix produced by pleomorphic sarcoma cells, is observed in this figure.

Microscopic Pathology

- The presence of osteoids and neoplastic bone, sometimes with neoplastic cartilage, is characteristic of this tumor.

- Most cases of extra-skeletal osteosarcoma are very similar to MFH, regardless of the presence of osteoids. In other words, the pleomorphic component of their sarcoma dominates the other components.
- There is a reverse zoning phenomenon, which means that unlike myositis ossificans fibrosis, the central region contains osteoids and is therefore calcified, and proliferation of atypical spindle cells is observed in the tumor periphery. (In ossified fibrous myositis, the mature area, which is calcified, is in the periphery).
- A variable number of benign and malignant multinucleated giant cells are also observed.
- They are often associated with foci of bleeding.

Treatment and Prognosis

- Treatment is similar to bone osteosarcoma.
- The prognosis of the disease is very bad. The five-year life expectancy of these patients is 52%.

Bad Prognosis

- Tumor size greater or equal to 5 cm was reported in a report as a poor prognosis.
- High mitotic index is associated with poor prognosis.

Good Prognosis

- The fibroblastic type in one report and the chondroblastic type in another report were considered a good prognosis.
- Extraosseous chondrosarcoma of mesenchymal type.

Definition

- Malignant cartilaginous tumor in soft tissue that consists of two components: sheets of mesenchymal cells.
- Primary and visual islands are well differentiated from hyaline cartilage.

Epidemiology

- The most common age is 15 to 35 years.
- Even congenital cases have been reported.
- M <F.

Common Site

- Head and neck, especially orbit.
- In the skull and spine.
- Lower limbs, especially the thighs.

Clinical Signs

- Pain, exophthalmos, blurred vision, and headache in orbital lesions.
- Vomiting, headache, various sensory and motor defects in skull and spine lesions.
- Painless mass with slow growth within the muscles in the lesion of the limbs.

Note

- Cases of bone mesenchymal chondrosarcoma metastasizing into soft tissue are similar to early soft tissue mesenchymal chondrosarcoma, so examination of the bone in soft tissue mesenchymal chondrosarcoma is recommended and necessary.

Imaging

- Soft tissue mass with a definite margin is observed on radiography with spot, filamentous or arcuate calcification due to calcification in cartilaginous areas.
- MRI: Dark in T1 and bright in T2.

Macroscopic Pathology

- Multiple mass of marginal lobules (with definite margin) with variable size (2.5 to 37 cm).
- The cutting surface is a mixture of soft gray-white fleshy tissue with foci of cartilage and bone with irregular size.
- Bleeding can occur, although it is much rarer than the myxoid type.
- Areas of necrosis may also be present.

Microscopic Pathology

- It consists of two histological areas.
- Part of the tumor is undifferentiated round, oval, or spindle-shaped cells.
- The other part consists of small nodules with a definite margin of hyaline cartilage with good differentiation and benign appearance, usually accompanied by calcification or ossification.
- The transformation of the histological view between the above two areas is quite sudden.

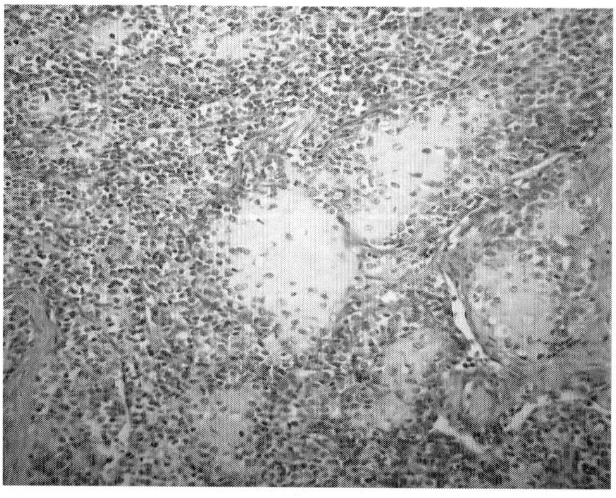

Figure 6-18. External bone mesenchymal chondrosarcoma. Its histological appearance consists of areas with small cells, and islands of hyaline cartilage. The vascular pattern of the tumor also seen.

Differential Diagnosis

- Small biopsy specimens with a needle biopsy that include only one of the zones of the tumor cause diagnostic problems, although the type of tumor, t-type obtained in a large biopsy does not have a diagnostic problem.
- If cartilaginous elements are not present, they may be mistaken with Ewing's Sarcoma/PENT, or low-grade synovial sarcoma, or malignant hemangiopericytoma.
- Hyaline cartilage foci help to differentiate chondrosarcoma from the above.

Treatment and Clinical Behavior

- Treatment includes extensive resection with radiotherapy or chemotherapy.
- 5-year survival is 55%.
- Metastasis is most common in the lungs.

EXTRAOSSEOUS CHONDROSARCOMA OF THE MYXOID TYPE

Definition

- Malignant cartilaginous tumors include cords or clumps of chondroblast-like cells located in the myxoid matrix.

Other Names

- Chondroid sarcoma (sarcoma).
- Tenosynovial sarcoma.

Epidemiology

- It is rare.
- It is most often observed in people over 35 years of age.
- The peak age is in the fifth or sixth decade.
- It is twice as common in men as in women.

Common Site

- Proximal limbs and girdle area, especially thighs and popliteal: 2/3 cases (similar to liposarcoma myxoid).
- It is more common in the lower extremities than in the upper extremities. About sixty percent of the cases occur in the lower extremities.

Clinical Signs

- Deep mass with slow growth.
- Has pain and tenderness in 1/3 of the cases.
- Bleeding inside the tumor or injury to large tumors may be observed.
- The duration of symptoms varies from a few weeks to several years. They are usually long-term symptoms.

Imaging

- Its symptoms are the same as all soft tissue sarcoma tumors. Pulmonary metastasis are usually observed in the early stages of the disease and are observed as countless marble lesions throughout the lung field (shape).

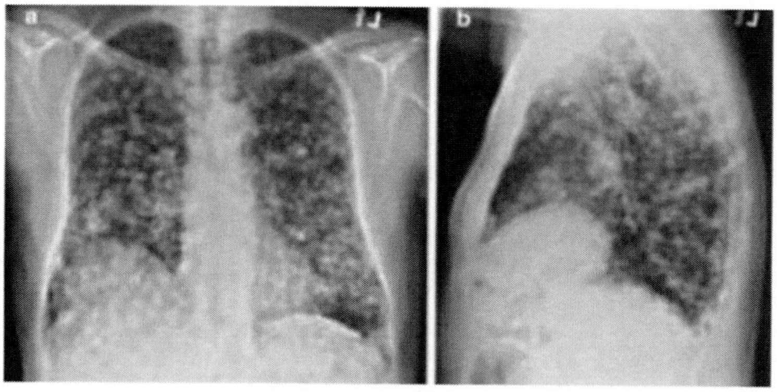

Figure 6-19. Pulmonary metastases in myxoid chondrosarcoma X-ray.

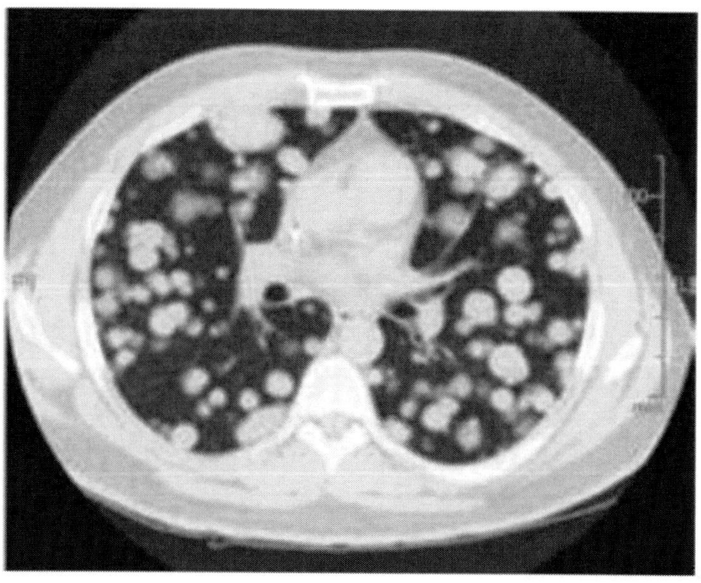

Figure 6-20. Pulmonary metastases in myxoid chondrosarcoma in CT-scan.

Macroscopic Pathology

- A mass with a definite border surrounded by a thick fibrous with false capsule In ovoid shape and the appearance of lobules with a soft to firm consistency.
- On the cutting surface, the gelatinous surface is gray to brown-tan.
- Tumor color depends on the amount of inside hemorrhage.
- Sometimes the bleeding is so extensive that it is mistaken with hematoma.
- Tumors with high cellularity have a fleshy appearance.
- Tumor size is usually 4 to 7 cm at the time of surgery. However, smaller sizes as well as larger than 15 cm have been observed.

Microscopic Pathology

- Multi-nodular pattern is evident at low power (small magnification).
- Nodules are made up of round to slightly elongated cells of the same size and shape that are separated by varying amounts of mucoid material.
- The small hyperchromatic nucleus and cytoplasm are observed as highly thin eosinophils.
- The cells are formed as false ropes, strands, or asymmetries that create a swollen appearance together.

Differential Diagnosis

- Parosteal chondrosarcoma: No myxoid component. It has extensive adhesions to the perichondrium or periosteum of the bone. It sometimes invades the lower cortex, causing irregularities on its outer surface.
- Myxoid liposarcoma: has a pattern of vascular networks. Typical lipoblasts, especially in the periphery
- There are tumor lobules.
- Unlike chondrosarcoma, it lacks pigmented mucin after hyaluronidase exposure.

Treatment and Clinical Behavior

- Wide resection with or without radiotherapy is the treatment for this tumor.
- Good results have been reported with radiotherapy and high-dose therapy (6000 cgy).
- Chemotherapy is not effective.
- The 5-year survival is 90%, which is much better than extracellular mesenchymal chondrosarcoma.
- Delayed recurrence and metastasis may occur.
- The rates of local recurrence and metastasis were 48% and 16%, respectively.
- Extra skeletal Ewing's sarcoma/PNET

History

- It was first reported in 1918 by Arthur Purdy Stoutt in a patient with round ulnar nerve tumor.

Epidemiology

- Most are under 30 years old. The age range in PNET is wider.

- It is slightly more common in men than women.
- No family relationship or relationship with environmental factors were found.

Site Involved

- Can be found anywhere.
- It is more common in deep soft tissue of the limbs.
- Common areas: Proximal thighs and buttocks, then proximal arms and shoulder.
- Tumors that are too close to the nerve can be associated with decreased nerve function.

Clinical Signs

- It is growing fast.
- It occurs as a deep mass.
- In the largest dimension it is 5 to 10 cm.
- Pain: observed in 1/3 of the cases.
- Progressive sensory and motor disorders can be observed if the peripheral nerves or spinal cord are involved.
- The patient's preoperative symptoms are less than the same as in all other Randsell sarcomas.
- Unlike neuroblastoma, catecholamine levels are normal.
- For diagnosis, Ct and PET MRI are performed routinely.

Macroscopic Pathology

- Multi-lobulated, soft and brittle.
- It is rarely larger than 10 cm.
- The surface of the cut is yellow, gray or tan gray.
- It is often associated with large areas of necrosis, bleeding, or cyst formation.
- Despite extensive necrosis, calcification is rare.

Microscopic Pathology

- Dense homogeneous accumulation of lobular round cells.
- The nucleus is all round or oval and 10 to 15 microns in diameter.
- CD99 Almost all round cell tumors in the differential diagnosis of ES / PNET can respond to CD99: lymphomas Merkel cell carcinoma, small cell carcinoma, rhabdomyosarcoma, mesenchymal chondrosarcoma, osteosarcoma.
- Cytogenetics: The most common chromosomal shift is T (11,22) (q24, q12), which is detected in 90% of the cases. This condition leads to the production of oncoproteins.

Treatment and Clinical Course

- The prognosis of ossifying Ewing and non-ossifying Ewing is the same in Western societies. In Japan, where Ewing is less prevalent, the extracellular type has a better prognosis.

CONGENITAL AND INFANTILE FIBROSARCOMA

Definition

- Infiltrative fibrosarcoma rarely metastasizes during infantile.

Epidemiology

- It is relatively rare.
- There are up to 1/3 cases exist at birth.
- In most cases, the tumor appears in first year of life.
- M> F (slightly)

Common Site

- The limbs are the main site of conflict. Especially distal to the knees and elbows.
- Head and neck, trunks are the next most common.

Clinical Signs

- Painless swelling or mass without tenderness with variable size from 1 to 20 cm.
- Tumor growth is very fast.

Imaging

- Soft tissue mass.
- Thickening of the cortex, bending deformity, and rarely extensive destruction of the underlying bone can be observed.
- Ultrasound and MRI help to diagnose congenital tumors in the uterus.

Macroscopic Pathology

- Size is variable.
- Ulcerative exophytic mass is observed in some patients.
- Most tumors have an indistinct margin. They are spindle or disc-shaped.
- They have a white-gray or pale pink appearance on the cutting surface.
- Large tumors may have necrosis or central hemorrhage or extensive myxoid or cystic changes.
- Transmission of t (12; 15) (p13; 125) is a characteristic feature of this tumor.

Microscopic Pathology

- They are similar to the adult types of this tumor.

- Sheets of dense, well-arranged spindle cells in the form of bundles or fascicles that give the appearance of herringbone.
- Nuclear pleomorphism is rare.
- The amount of mitosis from one area to another in the same tumor can vary.
- Tumors that contain a lot of collagen are similar to adult fibrosarcoma and are called desmoplastic type.
- Tumors containing low collagen are called medullary type.

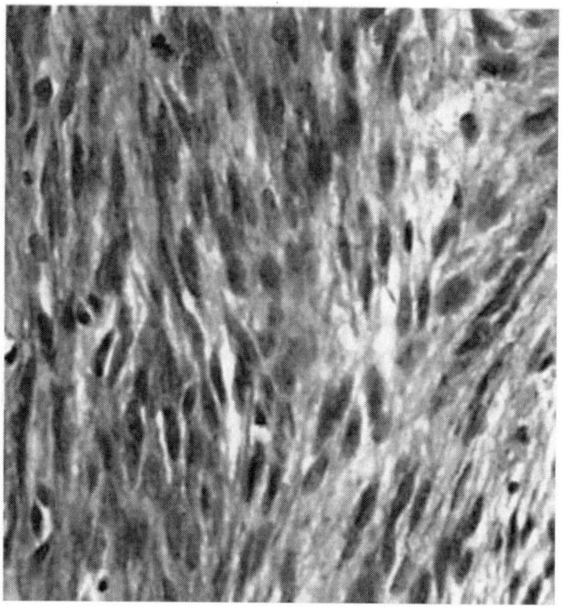

Figure 6-21. Congenital and infantile fibrosarcoma: Sheets of dense, well-arranged spindle cells in the form of bundles or fascicles that give the appearance of herringbone. Nuclear pleomorphism is rare.

Differential Diagnosis

- Infantile fibromatosis: Finding chromosomal abnormality t (12; 15) is in favor of congenital fibrosarcoma.

Treatment and Clinical Behavior

- Wide local excision is the main treatment.
- Preoperative chemotherapy reduces the size of the tumor and allows for more conservative surgery (some reports).
- Chemotherapy after surgery has also been successful (some reports).
- The value of radiotherapy is difficult to assess. Due to the risk of damage to the pediatrics physis in limb fibrosarcoma unless the radiotherapy field does not conclude the physis.
- Generally, treatment is surgical, and chemotherapy / radiotherapy in young people has to be used for non-surgical or recurrent metastatic cases.
- Congenital/infant type has a better prognosis than adult fibrosarcoma.
- Tumor cellularity, count (amount) of mitosis or extent of necrosis of the tumor, have no strong relationships with clinical behavior.

- There are reports that congenital/infant fibrosarcoma that is incompletely resected had no recurrence or metastasis for a long time. Cases of spontaneous regression have even been reported.
- There was no difference in patient age and tumor size and site of involvement in Tumors with recurrence in comparison to those without recurrence.

ABOUT THE AUTHORS

Babak Otoukesh, MD
Clinical Orthopedic Fellowship from Universitätsklinikum Bonn (UKB),
Orthopedic Surgeon at Department of Orthopedic Surgery,
Iran University of Medical Sciences in Rasoul-E-Akram hospital, Tehran, Iran
Email:babak.otoukesh@hotmail.com

Mehrdad Bahrabadi, MD
Assistant Professor of Orthopedic Surgery,
Musculoskeletal Tumor Fellowship,
Iran University of Medical Sciences, Tehran, Iran
Email: mehrdad.bahrabadi@gmail.com

Raphaelle Vialle, MD
Professeur des Universités - Praticien Hospitalier, Chef du Service de Chirurgie Orthopédique et Réparatrice de l'Enfant, Département Hospitalo-Universitaire MAMUTH "Maladies Musculo-Squelettiques et Innovations Thérapeutiques",
Hôpital Armand Trousseau, Université Pierre et Marie Curie, Paris, France
Email: raphael.vialle@aphp.fr

Shayan Hoseinzadeh, MD
Orthopedic Surgery Research Fellow,
Boston's Children Hospital, Harvard Medical School, Boston, US
Email: Shayan.hosseinzadeh@childrens.harvard.edu

Farnoosh Sedaghati, MD
Clinical and Anatomical Pathologist,
Iran University of Medical Sciences, Tehran, Iran
Email: sedaghati.farnoosh@gmail.com

Shayan Amiri, MD
Clinical Orthopedic Surgery Resident,
Bone and Joint Reconstruction Research Center,
Iran University of Medical Sciences, Tehran, Iran
Email: amiri.shayan23@gmail.com

INDEX

A

B

C

D

E

F

G

H

I

J

L

M

N

O

P

R

S

T

U

V

W